Pictures supplied by
Barnaby's: page 7 (top & bottom right)
Camera Press: pages 62, 64 (right)
Colour Sport: page 64 (left)
Mary Evans Picture Library: page 8 (left &
right)
Picturepoint: page 7 (left)
Syndication International: page 14
Transworld: page 6
Victoria & Albert Museum London
E. F. Burney: Elegant Establishment
for Young Ladies (detail): page 9
Cover and all other photographs:
Malcolm Scoular.

Text by: Sally-Anne Voak

Published by arrangement with
Marshall Cavendish Limited,
58 Old Compton Street,
LONDON W1V 5PA.

Library of Congress Catalog Card Number:
76-51537

ISBN 0-88365-391-5

Printed in Great Britain

Some of this material has appeared in the
publication. *The Natural Way to Keep in Shape*.

This volume is not to be sold outside the
USA and the Philippines.

Introduction

Everyone would like to be really fit and healthy, and the current trend for slender body contours and a trim outline, means that no-one can afford to be careless about eating the correct foods for health and energy.

Few people, however, recognize the need for exercise and to many, the very word makes them ache in every limb.

It need not be exhausting, and if you choose a properly planned exercise program to suit your life style it can become a regular part of your normal everyday life.

The Natural Way to Keep in Shape will provide you with the ideal start, with exercises and exercise programs for every part of your body. It will also explain simply and clearly how your body works, why it needs exercise and more important, all the benefits of a healthy way of life, good posture, relaxation and fitness. There are exercises for problem areas, streamline exercises, even exercises for those men (and lucky girls) who want to build up rather than trim down.

So start today and learn to enjoy the benefits of increased vitality and a trim and supple figure.

Contents

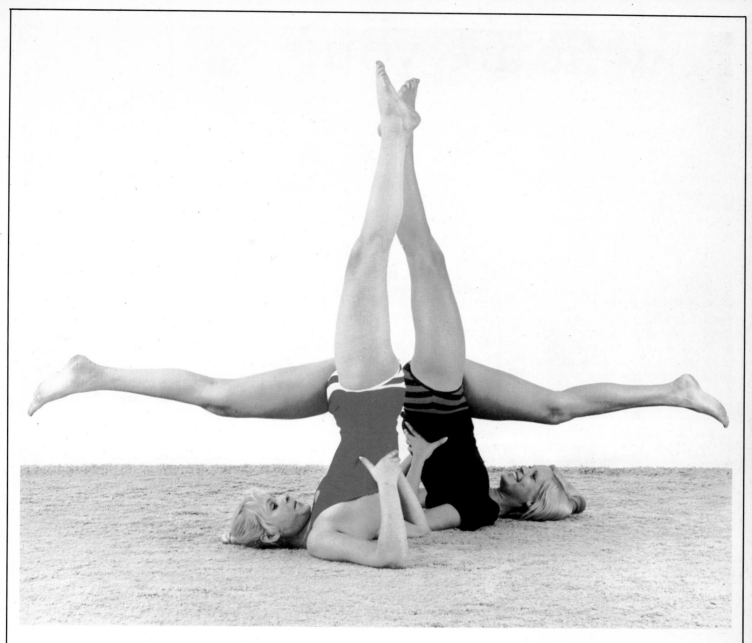

why exercise?

The man or woman who takes regular exercise will stay physically fit, retain youthful vigour and, perhaps most important to many people, keep a youthful shape. Good muscle tone is not, as some people fear, synonymous with bulging biceps or muscular thighs and most of the exercises given here are designed to keep you supple and make you look slimmer. While for those men (or skinny girls) who want to build themselves up we include a section on weight training.

To keep in good shape everyone needs a certain amount of exercise and, unfortunately, people are leading in-creasingly sedentary existences.

This means that you deliberately have to plan to include a daily exercise session, since everyday life no longer provides enough exercise.

Exercise is not just an overstated preoccupation of fitness fanatics; and it need not entail deep breathing by an open window in mid-winter, nor involve the use of cumbersome, expensive equipment.

In the following pages there is information about how your muscles work and why breathing and posture are important—all of which will help you to appreciate just how vital exercise is.

And there are exercises to suit everyone: planned exercise routines; exercises that take up little time, and those which will improve a problem area—ideal for anyone who has dieted carefully but not lost the desired number of inches from hips and waist. (Exercise is, of course, vital during and after a diet, for it helps to tone up flabby muscles—emphasizing your new, slimmer shape.)

Start doing some exercises every day and you will soon feel—and see—the benefits. Improved muscle tone—brought about by regular exercise—is visible in a more streamlined shape. And once you start exercising you become aware of your body and so correct bad posture habits, which again improves your shape. Finally, exercise will give you added energy and enthusiasm—because to be fitter means to to feel better.

1

how fit are you?

If you have never considered that you needed to take exercise just consider these few simple questions:

1. Do you sometimes go to bed mentally exhausted but find that you are unable to sleep?

2. Do you automatically ride up and avoid the stairs when you are visiting someone in an office or multi-storey building—even when they are only on the first or second floor?

3. If you can just manage to catch your train or bus by running for it do you make the effort—or do you wait for the next one to come along?

4. If you have to undertake some un-expected strenuous physical exercise such as mowing the lawn or decorating the spare room, do you feel aching and exhausted the next day?

5. Do you ever suffer from backache or headaches?

6. Are you dissatisfied with your figure?

7. Is your holiday the only time when you feel really rested and invigorated?

8. In the evenings, at the end of another tiring day, do you sit, slumped and exhausted, with just a vague feeling that you are not getting as much out of life as you should?

If the answer to only one of these questions is 'yes' then you are not 100 per cent fit, and you could benefit from a controlled programme of regular daily exercises.

If you want to feel fit—and you should —then you have to make up your mind to set aside a little time each day for exercise. You do not have to embark on a three-hour programme of physical jerks straight away. (Indeed, you will probably harm yourself if you do.) With the help of the gradual exercise plan in this book you can work up, at your own pace, to a programme which suits you.

Once you start to devote 10, 20 or 30 minutes a day to exercising you will begin to feel the benefits. You will feel less tired, more able to cope with the demands of a busy life and, miraculously, able to fit even more activities into each day. If you are young, you will stay feeling and looking young for longer. If you are older, you will start feeling truly youthful again. Those nagging everyday problems will fall into perspective and time-consuming minor aches and pains will become a thing of the past. If all this sounds too good to be true, just try it—you could be very surprised.

You may say you are conserving energy by not walking up the stairs or running for the bus. But is this an excuse? Do you use that energy for other things?

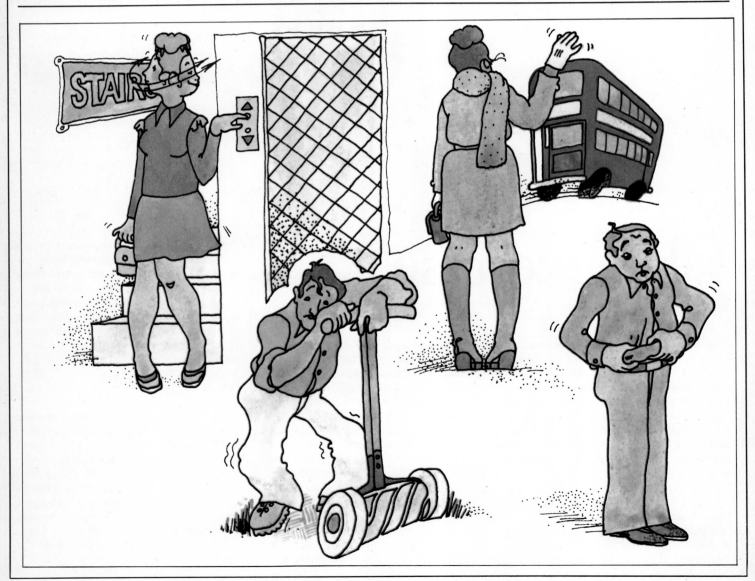

why you should exercise regularly

For most people, unfortunately, exercise comes way down the list of life's priorities—after work and leisure-time activities like socializing, eating and drinking. Yet doctors are constantly warning that today's largely sedentary existence, plus the effects of over-eating and lack of exercise are major causes of problems like heart trouble, nervous tension, muscular rheumatism, and circulatory and digestive upsets. These warnings usually go unheeded until it is too late, but just a regular half-hour stint of the correct exercises would be enough to ensure that you stayed in top form and led a long, active life.

Enjoy walking

How often do you go for a really long walk? If you are a car-owner, then the answer is probably never. Yet walking can benefit almost every muscle in the body—and it can be vastly enjoyable, too.

Try to allow yourself the luxury (and it is fast becoming one) of a walk every day. Walk part of the way to work for a change, or take an evening stroll around your neighbourhood. Get into the habit of walking to buy the Sunday papers instead of having them delivered or getting one of your children to buy them. Take your time, wear comfortable, well-fitting shoes and really enjoy yourself.

If you feel you need a stronger excuse for walking more often, then think seriously about taking up golf or getting a dog—or both. Once you are committed to a twice-weekly game or a daily constitutional with the dog the habit will probably stick.

Weatherwise, be brave. Walking in the rain can be fun if you are warmly dressed in a snug raincoat and boots. Children, particularly, like walking in the rain—and if there is a warm room and a hot bath waiting at home, the outing can do no harm. Even in hot weather a walk, taken slowly and steadily, can be enjoyable.

While you walk, think about posture and movement. Do not hunch your shoulders, drag your feet or amble along. Walk briskly, in an upright position with your arms swinging naturally. If you must carry heavy parcels, it is better to distribute them evenly between two baskets or bags (one in each hand), than to hump one big load.

What exercise can do for your figure

Exercise alone will not make you lose weight. What it will do is to tighten up slack muscles and tone up your body after dieting. Many people find that regular exercise helps to maintain a steady weight level—once they stop, the pounds pile up. If the prospect of exercising every day for the rest of your

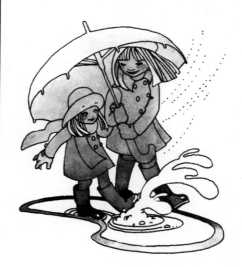

life sounds a bit gloomy, cheer up—it can be fun, too. Think of exercise as a streamlining treatment for your figure. In conjunction with a good low-calorie diet, it can do wonders for your shape.

What exercise can do for your health

Regular exercise can help you achieve a peak of physical fitness. That peak will obviously vary from individual to individual (a shorthand typist requires less stamina than a wrestler, for example), but in every case it means that the body is more able to resist disease. Even comparatively minor illnesses like the common cold are less likely to strike the person who is physically fit. And if you exercise regularly you will be vital and energetic for longer—keeping good health into middle age and beyond. If you are young this may not seem particularly important now, but remember that modern medicines and scientific developments are keeping man alive for longer—so why not be fit enough to enjoy the bonus of a contented, active retirement?

What exercise can do for your work

The most efficient businessmen are often those who take regular time off for exercise. There is a sound reason for this. Physical fitness means increased working efficiency—whether the job is sedentary or manual. If you are fit you find work less tiring and more rewarding. Working for 16 hours a day with just the odd break for a sandwich may be laudable—but in the long term it is unlikely to be in the best interests of the company or the employee. There is little point in working so hard that you are forced to take time off later when illness strikes.

What exercise can do for your family life

Physical fitness helps to give you energy to spare, so that you can really enjoy life with your family. Instead of spending weekends sitting indoors, you will have the strength and inclination to go on outings to the country, picnics by the sea or sight-seeing trips to the city. Just when your children are at their most demanding you will be able to keep up with them without tiring. Sadly, many parents seem to lose touch with their offspring simply because they feel too physically exhausted to cope with energetic youngsters. At weekends they send the children off to play with friends while they 'relax' by sitting at home. But regular exercise can make you feel you want to take up new hobbies, tackle new tasks, and do things as a family again.

Sudden exercise can be dangerous

Remember that sudden, strenuous exercise after very little can be extremely dangerous—particularly for those with a weak heart condition. If you feel you really must mow the lawn, then do not tackle it too strenuously if you have spent the last month or two sitting down all day and relaxing all evening. At best, you will feel tired and achey the next day—at worst, you could strain a muscle.

who is the fittest of them all?

Fitness is very difficult to define precisely. A weight-lifter with bulging biceps and abnormally strong abdominals may be able to lift 100 kilograms without flinching—but he may not be at a peak of physical fitness. Muscles developed to an unnatural degree are not necessarily healthy muscles, and the bandages many weight-lifters and wrestlers wear around their wrists and ankles prove this point.

At the other end of the weight-scale, a short, thin bank clerk could be described as 'fit' if he can cope adequately with all the physical and mental demands of the life he leads without aches, pains or ill-health.

The key to the answer to the fitness question lies in the life you lead. You should be in peak condition to tackle your everyday tasks, with a little in reserve to cope with any unexpected extra effort. Measure your fitness rating against the questions below.

Physical strength

Firstly, what kind of physical strength is required for your life? Do you have to carry heavy shopping, dig the garden, unload packing cases, push a baby-carriage, dig trenches in the road or drive a large vehicle? There is no point in developing the rippling muscles of a road-digger if your life is spent pounding a typewriter. But, if you enjoy gardening at weekends, then you need reserves of physical strength to cope with the extra exertion. Although men, generally, do need to be stronger than women some feminine tasks require muscular strength: lifting a healthy toddler, pushing a pram and carrying shopping all day demand more effort than sitting behind a cashier's window at a bank!

Stamina

Can you stand the pace of your life without tiring? Does the sudden effort of running for a bus reduce you to a gasping state of near collapse? For most people it is unnecessary and impractical to develop the stamina of an Olympic long-distance runner. But it is necessary to be able to enjoy a

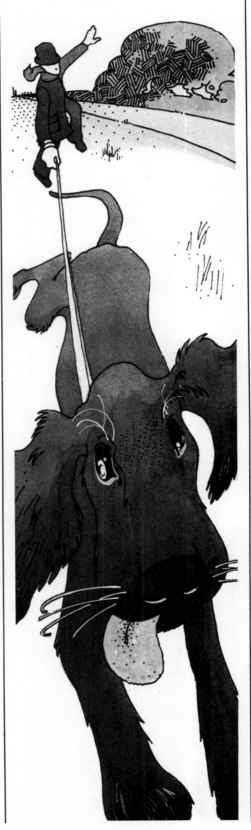

long country walk, for example, without suffering from short breath and a pounding heart after the first two miles. Measure your performance against the last test of stamina that you had to endure. How did you shape up? Were you exhausted? Were you taken aback because your companion, or your dog, had more stamina than you did?

Vitality

Do you enjoy your life? Does a sudden invitation or an unexpected visit by friends throw you into a state of tiredness and gloom, or do you manage to find reserves of vitality even after a tiring day? Only television and cabaret stars need a constant stream of jokes and untapped *joie-de-vivre*—but you should have enough energy to face life with enthusiasm. New challenges, in work or social life, should be welcomed. If you have started avoiding parties, people, tasks—then you are not fit.

Concentration

Can you apply yourself to a task with complete concentration, or does your mind wander? Perhaps your academic days are far behind you and it is unnecessary to apply yourself for hours to a complicated mathematical problem, but you may still have household accounts to do, or documents to study. You should be able to do this without fidgeting or worrying about problems, children, money, etc., at the same time. This ability to concentrate and separate thoughts into conveniently-sized packages, and to deal with problems one at a time, is all part of being well-adjusted to the life you lead. If your worries become a jumble of insurmountable problems which seem to be weighing down on you, then getting fit can actually help you to reorganize your life.

Relaxation

Can you relax? Can you put worries out of your mind and truly relax your body? Can you sit quietly and calmly, without outside stimuli, just for a few moments? If you cannot relax or sleep properly, if you wake up in the mornings exhausted, then you are not fit. If you can do these things, then that weight-lifter is probably nowhere near as fit as you are.

Fitness shows in your face, your figure and your approach to life. If you are not in good shape you may be unable to forget your worries and enjoy yourself.

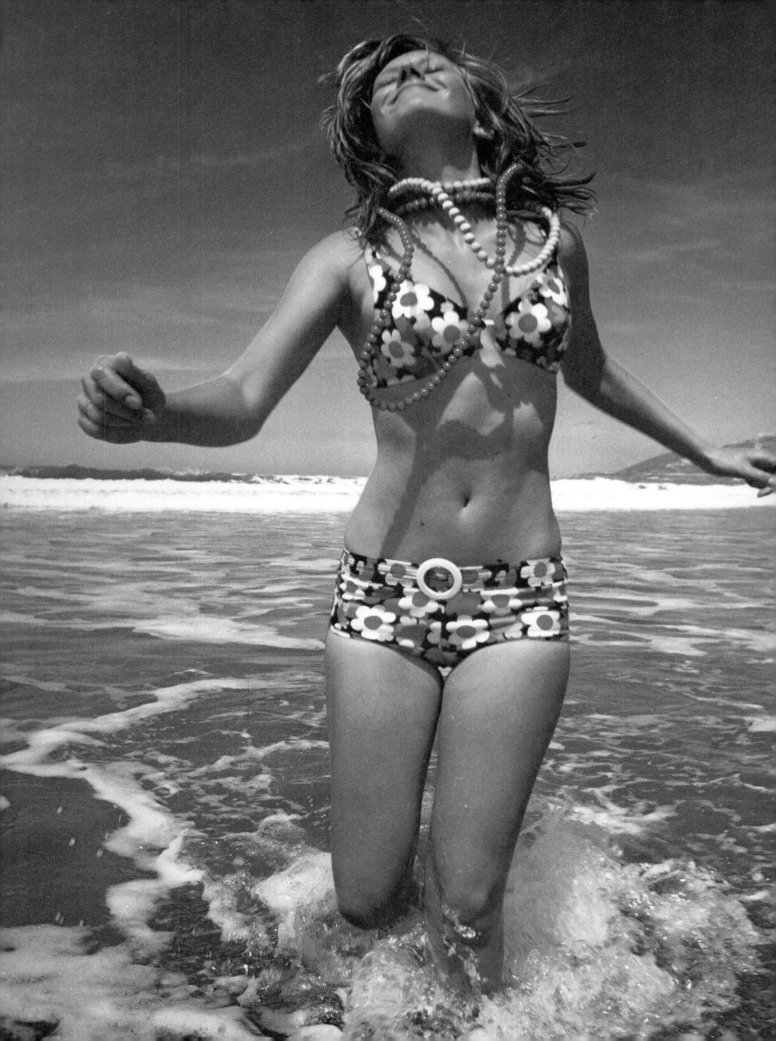

exercise and the life you lead

To a very large extent, the kind of controlled exercises you need are governed by the sort of work you do. If, for example, you spend eight hours every day typing, the muscles which control your fingers and the Wrist Extensors will get plenty of exercise already. (See pages 76-77 for a chart which explains the major muscle groups and the jobs they do.) However, while you are sitting typing the Buttock Group (which includes the Gluteus Maximus, Gluteus Medius, Gluteus Minimus,) and the Abductors (outside thigh) will be in a constant state of relaxation and if your posture is bad then the Trapezius and Rhomboids (back and shoulder muscles) will be lax too. Your daily exercise programme should, therefore, include movements which give these muscles work to do.

On the other hand, if you are a professional football player, then the Calves, Hamstring Group, Buttock Group and Quadriceps Femoris (front thigh) will be getting exercise—while your Biceps, Triceps and Wrist Extensors may be getting very little.

Muscle development is very closely linked with professional work. The main problems of people in sedentary jobs (secretarial, managerial, assembly-line work, accountancy, journalism, etc.,) are flabby muscles in the stomach, buttocks, and thighs—often accompanied by round or hunched shoulders. Even people who stand at work have their problems: waitresses constantly stooping develop rounded shoulders, sales girls get fallen arches, and heavy manual workers find that the strength they develop in their arms leaps way ahead of that developed in their back. By far the commonest problem is, however, that of the sedentary worker. He or she spends most of each day sitting down—at a desk or on an assembly line all day; in a car, bus or train to travel home; at a table to eat and then, finally, in a comfortable chair to relax. Even before planning a regular exercise routine, several steps can be taken to give the unused muscles more work to do—and so lessen the chances of 'sedentary workers' sag'.

Posture

While you are working, it is important to sit up straight, holding your abdominal muscles in and your shoulders back. (See the isometric exercises on pages 80-84—they will help to control any round-shouldered droop.)

Chair

Make sure your chair is the right height for the job. It is surprising how many workers go through life sitting day after day on a chair which is too low or too high to enable them to work comfortably. If you have to hunch yourself over your papers your muscles are bound to sag. Make sure the chair is comfortable—but hard. Buttock muscles which have nothing to resist against will sag alarmingly. Many an outsize typist's rear owes its existence to a large squashy cushion on her chair! And exactly the same rules apply for chairs at home. Do not sit in a soft armchair every evening; choose a straight-backed chair instead.

Travel

Choose a car which suits your shape. If you travel by car for several hours a day, it makes sense to be comfortable. A big man hunched up inside a tiny car for two hours a day is quite likely to develop a permanent stoop. Travelling time provides an excellent opportunity for isometric exercises (see pages 80-84), but if you are driving, you must, of course, concentrate on the road.

Lunch hour

Use your midday break for some pleasant, gentle exercise. Instead of eating in a canteen or restaurant, take a packed lunch to work with you and spend some time walking. Even if you are very busy this is a good idea. A short walk can often help to put office problems into perspective—and it can help you to keep physically fit.

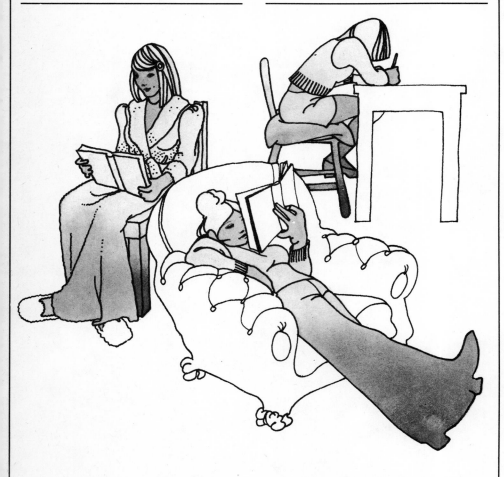

If you have a sedentary job or have business lunches your exercise needs will differ from those of a road-digger.

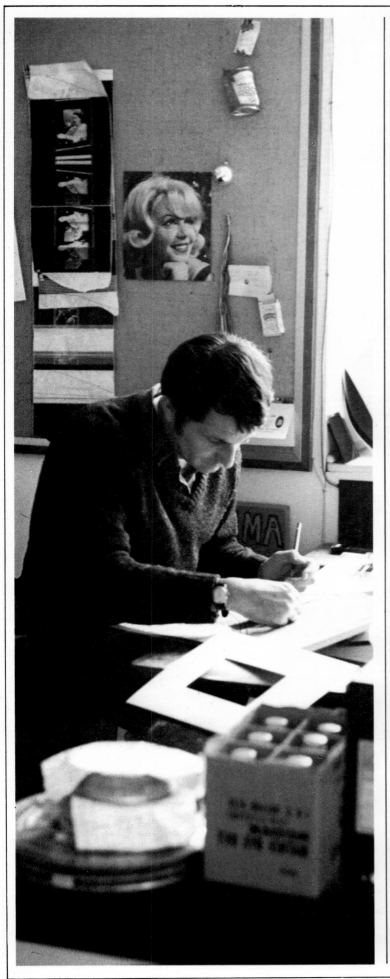

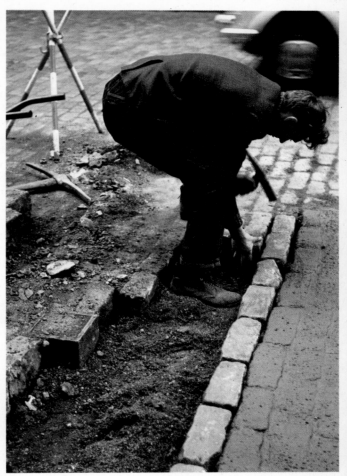

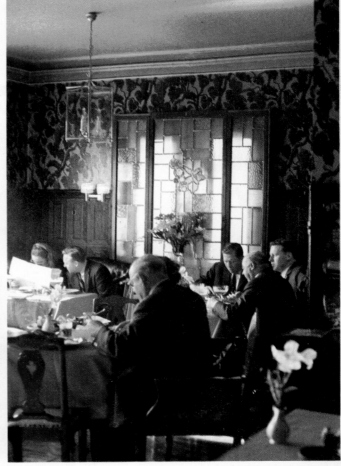

7

good posture matters

'Come along, don't slouch—let's see some straight backs and shoulders.' These are familiar words from school or army days, and most people hearing them took little or no notice. But those nagging commands to 'sit up straight, there!' were vitally important.

Without good posture, the organs of the body cannot work properly or, in the case of children, even develop properly. If only it had been explained exactly why posture mattered so much, one might have been a little more receptive to the idea of walking, sitting and standing correctly. There are excellent reasons for remembering to straighten your back and shoulders.

Childhood development In children, bones, muscles and organs are still growing. If posture is bad, this growth may be inhibited or may develop incorrectly. If, for example, the shoulders sag forward the chest will be cramped and the lungs unable to expand fully. Intake of oxygen will be limited and tiredness, lack of energy and bad resistance to disease may result. Unfortunately, too, sagging shoulders in childhood become a habit which is carried through into adult life—particularly if the child goes on to take up a sedentary job.

Digestion If the stomach and intestines are cramped because the spine is not being held upright food will not be 'processed' smoothly and indigestion will often result. (Eating meals sitting cramped in an armchair in front of a television is almost certain to produce acute indigestion.)

Backache If you walk with your head poked forward, there is a permanent strain on the muscles at the back of the neck and in the upper back. This often results in painful backache which could easily have been avoided with good posture.

Hip joints Walking with a 'wiggle' may be fashionable but it is not healthy. The pelvic girdle (band joining the hip bones) should always be kept as firm as possible and not allowed to wobble from side to side. Constant wobbling may loosen the joints between backbone and girdle, causing strained muscles and even arthritis.

Feet Walking with toes pointing outwards may cause swollen joints and even corns on the little toes. Cold feet, chilblains and hard skin are often the result of poor circulation caused by bad posture and stance—and using foot muscles wrongly. These bad walking habits, together with overweight and

ill-fitting shoes, can cause very painful foot conditions.

Physical tiredness If you are physically worn out at the end of the day, yet have not had any real exercise, bad posture could be the cause. If the body is not held correctly, your muscles have to do extra 'work' to keep it upright and, naturally, find the extra strain tiring. People in sedentary jobs, particularly, may find that they feel aching and tired after 3 or 4 hours spent writing or typing. Improving posture can often remove the problem completely.

Appearance If you sag you will look unattractive and lumpish—if you stand or sit well you immediately look slimmer and brighter. There is sound sense behind the old advice that at job interviews one should sit up straight.

Lift with ease

When you are going to lift anything— a piece of furniture, a suitcase or even

Machines to improve posture without effort have always been popular. One contraption claimed to make an ill-developed girl as straight as a lifeguardsman (left) while in 1892 this home gymnasium (below) was advertised.

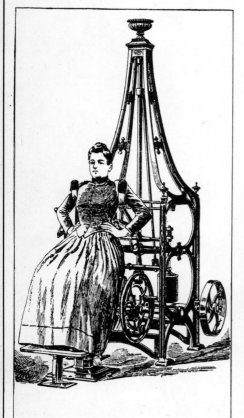

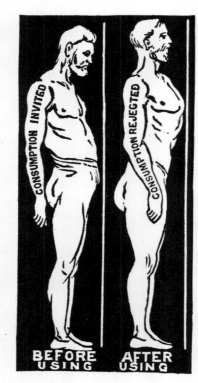

BEFORE USING   AFTER USING

a child—be careful to lift it in the right way and avoid pulling your back muscles. Never bend from your hips, but keep your back straight and bend at the knees. When you have a secure grip straighten your legs slowly and try not to bend forward. If you feel yourself losing balance put the weight down and start again.

How to improve your posture

Follow the simple rules given below and you will look better and feel better too.

Are you sitting comfortably?
Always make sure that your chair and table are at the correct heights. Your knees should fit comfortably under the table and your hands should touch the table-top without any unnecessary bending forward from the waist. A hard chair is usually more comfortable for longer than a soft one, and it is certainly better for your buttock muscles. Sit like this:
1. Press your buttocks against the back of the chair.
2. Press your thighs evenly on the seat of the chair with the hip-joint forming a right angle.
3. Hold your backbone comfortably upright—and if the back of the chair does not coincide with this position then do not lean on it.
4. Rest your feet flat on the floor (do not cross your ankles or knees) with the knee and ankle joints forming right angles.

Standing straight
Give some conscious thought to the way you stand; try to catch yourself in bad standing positions. In time, good posture will become a habit. Stand like this:
1. Balance your weight evenly on both feet.
2. Contract your buttock muscles to pull in your seat.
3. Hold in your abdominal muscles.
4. Hold your pelvic girdle evenly, hips on the same level. Do not tip it forward or backward.
5. Stretch your body upwards and hold yourself comfortably.
6. Keep your shoulders down and back and, above all, relaxed.
7. Hold your arms loosely by your sides.
8. Now imagine a straight line drawn from your left ear to the ground. It should pass through your neck, shoulder joint, elbow, hand, hip joint, knee and the front of your left ankle. (Check this in front of a long mirror.)

Walking tall
Watch your reflection in shop windows —are you walking properly? An elegant, relaxed walking posture is vital for good looks, and for good health. Walk like this:
1. Keep the same basic position as for standing.
2. Now tilt your body slightly forward as you change your weight from the back to the front foot.
3. Point your toes forward—not out to the side or inwards. Keep the weight mainly on the outside of the feet.
4. Lift your heels off the ground as you walk. (Do not exaggerate this but do not drag your feet either.)
5. Swing your arms gently as you walk. If it helps, chant silently to yourself as you go along: walk tall, back straight, head up, shoulders back, chest out, stomach in, seat under, swing each leg from the hip.

This torturous-looking piece of Regency appartus (below) was used to correct deportment and, probably, to produce a fashionable swan-like neck.

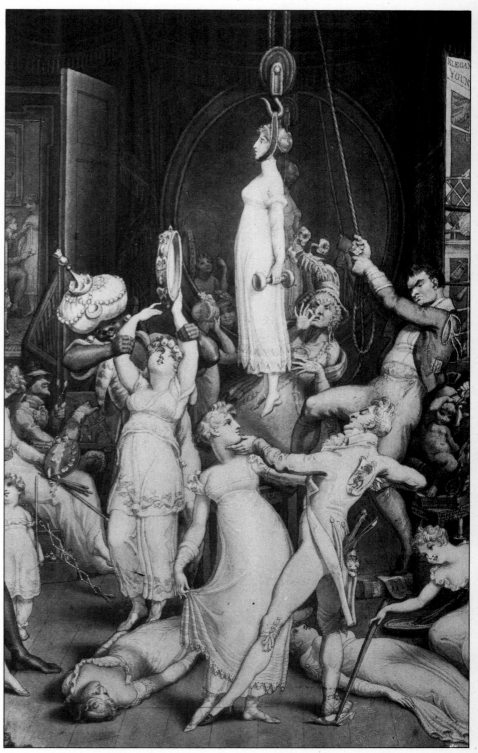

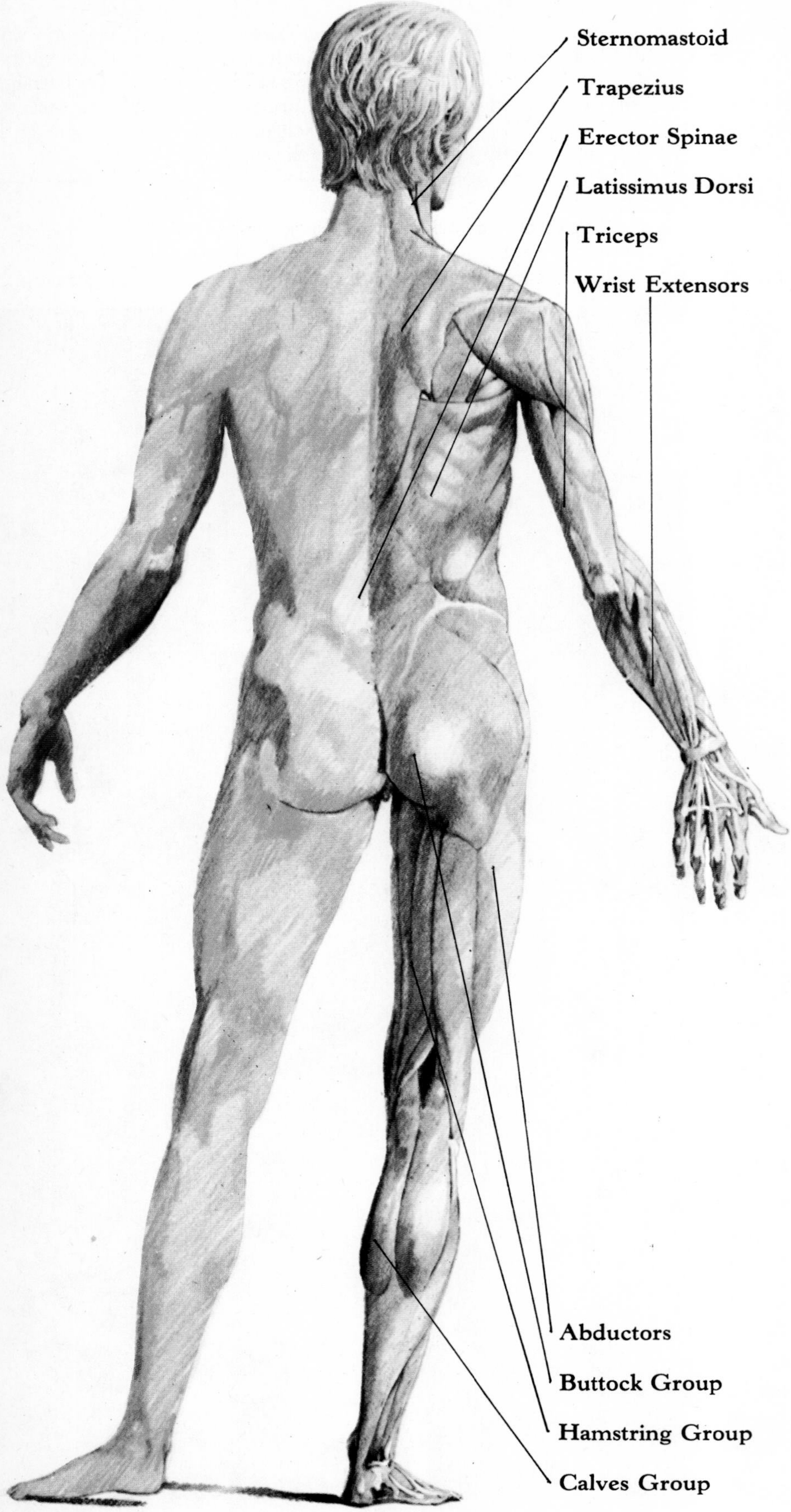

all about muscles

Sternomastoid

Trapezius

Erector Spinae

Latissimus Dorsi

Triceps

Wrist Extensors

Abductors

Buttock Group

Hamstring Group

Calves Group

What are they?

Over half the human body is composed of muscle fibres—fibres which control every single movement we make. Eating, breathing, talking, running, drinking and living itself would all be impossible without muscles. Muscles pull your mouth upwards in a smile if you are happy, make your fingers move to pick up a cup of coffee, and your legs move to run for the bus. Bad muscle tone, therefore, affects your whole life.

What are they made of?

Muscles are made of three different kinds of tissue: **cardiac** muscle tissue (found in the heart—the most important muscle in our body), **smooth** muscle tissue which lines the walls of intestines and arteries, and **striped** muscle tissue which forms the skeletal muscles like those of the arms and legs. Under a microscope, striped muscle tissue looks like lots of tiny cylindrical fibres, bound by connective tissue and encased in a fibrous sheath.

What do they do?

The smooth-tissued **involuntary** muscles have a happy knack of getting on with things alone. The intestine muscles take care of food once it has been eaten, the arterial wall muscles pump blood from the heart and the heart itself just goes on quietly beating without any conscious message from the brain.

The **voluntary** muscles (which are most concerned with exercising) need stimulus from the nervous system before they can contract and set a movement in motion. You may not consider that you send a message to your feet every time you take a step, or even consciously think about laughing or crying—but your brain does anticipate these actions, and sends the right message to the appropriate muscle.

How do they do it?

The muscles are attached to the skeletal bones by short, tough tendons. On receiving a 'message' from the brain the muscles contract, pulling the appropriate part of the skeletal frame with them—the tendons prevent them from coming adrift. The frame itself moves smoothly with the help of the joints between the bones—ball-and-socket joints like the hips and shoulders; hinge joints like the elbow and knee; gliding joints like those that link the vertebrae. The muscles are kept in a constant state of partial contraction, ready for the full contraction which comes with that message from the brain. This state is called 'muscle tone'—good muscle tone means strength, firmness and elasticity —and that means fitness.

What makes good muscle tone?

The right kind of regular exercise keeps muscles in a constant state of readiness, so that any sudden necessary activity can be coped with without creaks and aches. Rest and relaxation are also important, because emotions like anxiety, fear, overwork and sleeplessness can contract the muscles more than the limit required for perfect tone. This brings a feeling of tension and can lead to backaches, headaches and other uncomfortable symptoms. Very slack muscle tone, on the other hand, usually means that extra exertion is difficult, or painful, and it can also lead to pockets of fat being formed around the slack muscle.

The musculature of a man and a woman (left and right) are identical—
a woman's more rounded hips, etc. are due to extra layers of fatty tissue.
The muscles identified here are those discussed in the chart on the following two pages, where we also tell you how to exercise each muscle.

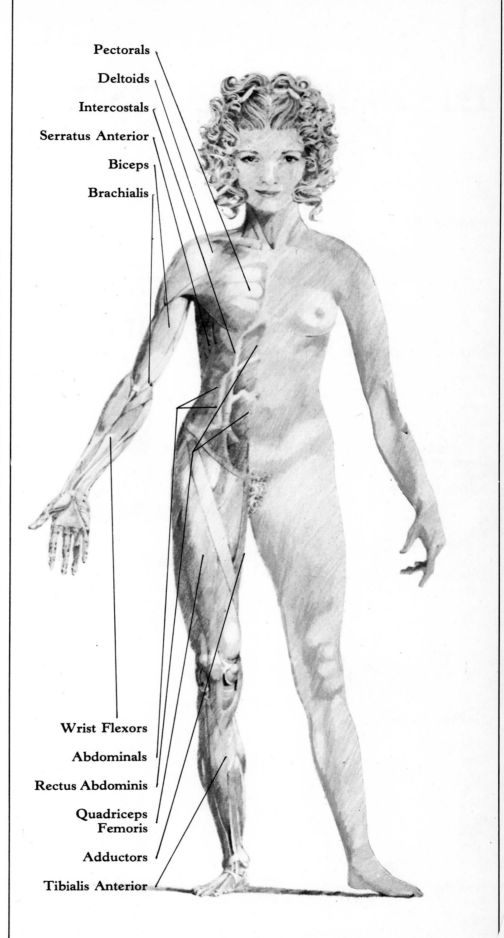

Pectorals
Deltoids
Intercostals
Serratus Anterior
Biceps
Brachialis

Wrist Flexors
Abdominals
Rectus Abdominis
Quadriceps Femoris
Adductors
Tibialis Anterior

the major muscles and muscle groups

Name: Sternomastoid

Where they are:
Each side of the neck.

What they do:
Each side acts independently to bend the head sideways and turn the head. And they both act together to bend the head on to the chest.

How they should be exercised:
By head bending and rotation.

Name: Trapezius

Where it is:
This is a triangular shaped muscle across the back of the neck and shoulders.

What it does:
Draws shoulders together and downwards and generally acts as a brace for the shoulders. Bad tone in the Trapezius can aggravate 'dowager's hump' and round shoulders. The Trapezius takes a lot of strain if you sit hunched over a desk or typewriter for long hours.

How it should be exercised:
Shoulder circling and controlled arm movements.

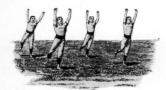

Name: Deltoids

Where they are:
Over the top of the shoulders, covering the shoulder joints like epaulettes.

What they do:
Raise the arms up to shoulder level sideways and, in conjunction with other muscles, help rotate the arms and raise them to the front and back.

How they should be exercised:
By any arm-raising movement or lifting weights. Sports like gymnastics, climbing, tennis or boxing are also good for for the Deltoid muscles.

Name: Latissimus Dorsi

Where it is:
This is a broad muscle which stretches across the back into the back of the arms.

What it does:
Helps to draw arms down and back and to rotate them. Also pulls trunk up towards static arms (as in rope-climbing).

How it should be exercised:
By pulling the arms down and back, preferably against resistance. Sports like rowing and climbing are good. too.

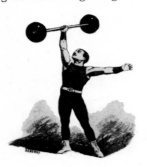

Name: Brachialis

Where they are:
Front of the upper arms, across the joints.

What they do:
Help to flex the arm in conjunction with the Biceps.

How they should be exercised:
By arm-bending against some kind of resistance—weight-lifting is good. Activities like digging and shovelling earth also provide good exercise for these muscles.

Name: Biceps

Where they are:
Top of the front of the upper arms.

What they do:
Turn the hands palm upwards to bend the arms.

How can they be exercised:
In the same way as the Brachialis.

Name: Triceps

Where they are:
Back of the upper arms.

What they do:
Straighten the elbows.

How they should be exercised:
By pushing arms against resistance, and by throwing, punching, pushing. Sports like cricket (bowling), baseball (pitching), shot-put, javelin, boxing and fencing develop and strengthen them.

Name: Wrist Flexors

Where they are:
On the fronts of the forearms.

What they do:
Help bend the palms of the hands towards you.

How they should be exercised:
By hand-gripping and pushing the wrists forwards. Sports like golf, tennis, bowling, squash and badminton are all good for these muscles.

Name: Wrist Extensors

Where they are:
Back of forearms.

What they do:
Pull the back of the hand away from you.

How they should be exercised:
Fist-clenching and gripping and handstands.

Name: Pectorals

Where they are:
Upper chest.

What they do:
Help to draw the arms across the body and rotate the arms inwards. In women they support the breasts.

How they should be exercised:
By strong resistance of the hands against an immovable object. By clasping your hands in front of your chest and pulling outwards.

Name: Serratus Anterior

Where they are:
Sides of the upper rib cage.

What they do:
Help you push with your arms.

How they should be exercised:
By pushing against resistance, or by everyday activities like mowing the lawn, carpet-sweeping, vacuum-cleaning.

Name: Intercostals

Where they are:
Between the ribs, in two distinct layers.

What they do:
Help you breathe by raising and lowering the ribs as you inhale and exhale.

How they should be exercised:
By deep, regular breathing.

Name: Abdominals

Where they are:
The Abdominal group (which includes internal and external Obliques and Transversalis) forms a muscular 'corset' three layers thick between the diaphragm and pelvis.

What they do:
Bend the trunk from side to side, rotate it and support the stomach, Strong abdominals give a flat, firm stomach.

How they should be exercised:
By bending and twisting the trunk. Dancing, gymnastics and sports involving throwing can also help.

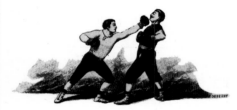

Name: Rectus Abdominis

Where they are:
They extend down the middle of the Abdominals to the pubic bone.

What they do:
They bend the trunk forward.

How they should be exercised:
By bending the trunk forward. Sports involving forward movements such as rowing are good, too. Sit-ups and leg-raises are the exercises which help strengthen these muscles.

Name: Erector Spinae

Where they are:
They extend each side of the whole length of the spinal column.

What they are:
Help the spine to move smoothly and keep the trunk erect.

How they should be exercised:
By back-arching or raising the trunk from a bent forward position.

Name: Buttock Group

Where they are:
This is the name given to the group of muscles which extend all over the seat.

What they do:
Pull the thighs sideways and pull them backwards. They also revolve the legs and some of the muscles in the group help raise the trunk from a stooping position. Firm buttock muscles are vital for a trim figure.

How they should be exercised:
By raising legs backwards (see exercise on page 121) and by contraction. Most fairly strenuous sports and activities can help—swimming, dancing, running, walking, etc.

Name: Hamstring Group

Where they are:
Rear of thighs.

What they do:
Bend the knees and help to rotate them outwards and extend the legs backwards. The Hamstring group are particularly vulnerable—daily exercise such as walking and sitting simply do not exercise them enough and a sudden strain can cause damage.

How they should be exercised:
Toe-touching and leg-stretching.

Name: Quadriceps Femoris

Where they are:
Front of thighs.

What they do:
Extend the knees and bend the hips.

How they should be exercised:
Leg straightening and kicking movements. Games like football, rugby, running, walking and climbing are all good.

Name: Tibialis Anterior

Where they are:
Front of lower legs.

What they do:
Raise toes and feet up and towards you and turn the feet inwards.

How should they be exercised:
Foot bending and circling and turning feet up and inwards.

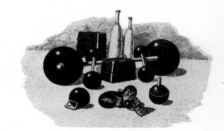

Name: Calves Group

Where they are:
Back of lower legs.

What they do:
Raise heels and point toes downwards.

How they should be exercised:
Heel-raising and toe-pointing, standing on tiptoes, walking, running, jumping, dancing.

Name: Adductors

Where they are:
Insides of the thighs.

What they do:
Pull upper legs inwards.

How they should be exercised:
Fat often accumulates around these muscles because they are so unused. They can be exercised by pushing legs tightly together—riding and swimming (breast stroke) can also help.

Name: Abductors

Where they are:
Outsides of the thighs. These muscles insert into the soft tissue of the lower thigh and therefore have no bony connection. That is why fat is so easily accumulated on the outer thigh.

What they do:
Carry the leg outwards, and rotate it inwards.

How they should be exercised:
By walking and running, always keeping the feet pointing forwards.

take a deep breath

Breathing is the basic activity that triggers off all the complicated mechanisms of the body, and so keeps us alive. Basically, the respiratory system's job is to bring air and blood into close contact with each other so that oxygen can pass from the air into the blood, and carbon dioxide can diffuse from the blood into air.

It is oxygen which starts off the chain of reaction known as body metabolism —without it, we cannot survive.

Organs of the respiratory system and what they do

Nose. The nose provides the openings through which the air can enter the body. The tiny hairs in the nostrils help to remove dirt and impurities from the air before it enters the lungs. The nasal passages warm the air to body-temperature. Even the nasal fluid helps by trapping and killing bacteria. The nose also provides a sense of smell and gives the voice resonance.

Throat. The throat directs food from the mouth into the food canal, directs air from the nose into the windpipe and allows air to enter and leave the middle ears, thus enabling hearing to take place.

Windpipe and bronchial tubes. These are the air passages. The windpipe leads from the throat into the chest cavity, where it divides into two branches—the bronchial tubes. Together, these passages warm, moisten and clean the air before it enters the lungs. Inside the lungs the tubes divide again and again into smaller tubes.

Lungs. The lungs provide a large surface over which the air and blood can be brought into contact, oxygen passing from the air into the blood and carbon dioxide from the blood into the air. The 'elastic' walls of the lungs allows them to expand—to hold large quantities of the air drawn into the body— and to contract—to expel the used air. (The capacity of the lungs is really amazing. If all the 'wrinkles' in the tissue of the two lungs were smoothed out they would cover an area equal to half the area of a tennis court.) Really deep, regular breathing means that the maximum amount of oxygen can be extracted from the air. Shallow, irregular breathing means that a patchy, irregular supply of oxygen is absorbed into the blood-stream.

How the lungs work

Breathing in. As the lungs expand, air is pushed in from the outside. To enable expansion to take place a layer of muscles between the ribs contracts, lifting the ribs upwards and outwards. Meanwhile, the muscles of the diaphragm also contract, making the diaphragm flatter and elongated in shape and thus deepening the chest cavity. Because the lungs expand, the pressure of the air already inside them is lower than that outside the body—therefore air is naturally pushed into the lungs through the nose and air passages.

Breathing out. A different layer of muscles between the ribs contracts, pulling the ribs downwards and inwards to their original positions and deflating the lungs in the process. Meanwhile

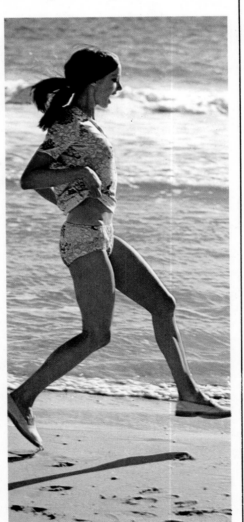

the diaphragm muscles relax, making the chest cavity smaller. Thus the air is forced out through the air passages.

Capacity. Inflating the whole 'half tennis court' area of the lungs would obviously be impossible because of the limitations of the rib-cage, but the lungs can hold a very large volume of air when fully expanded—something in the region of 4 litres. In normal breathing about $\frac{1}{10}$ litre of air is actually inhaled, and in deep breathing the capacity increases to about $2\frac{1}{2}$ litres.

Rate. The normal adult breathing rate is about 15 breaths a minute, and this is increased when exercise is being taken. It is vital to breathe in and out correctly when exercising. You will notice that breathing instructions are given with each exercise described later on; do follow these instructions carefully. If you hold your breath because you are concentrating on the exercise you restrict the supply of oxygen to the blood-stream. And if you breathe in the wrong place your ribs may be pulling against the exercise (that is, you may be breathing in, thus lifting your ribs upwards, while the movement of the exercise is pushing your ribs downwards) and the whole movement will become difficult and painful.

To help lungs to expand fully, and make you aware of good breathing
Stand straight, preferably by an open window, with your arms by your sides. Now exhale fully. Slowly raise your heels from the ground, lifting arms out to the sides and up above your head as you do so—breathe in slowly at the same time. Now slowly lower heels and arms, exhaling fully at the same time.
Repeats. Breathe regularly for a few seconds, then repeat once.

To help clear nasal passages, relieve headaches and aid good breathing
Clasp the bridge of your nose with the first two fingers of your right hand. Now press the back of your right thumb against your right nostril to close it completely. Inhale slowly through your left nostril to a count of six, close left nostril with the fourth finger of your right hand (still keeping thumb firmly pressed against your right nostril). Retain air for a count of six, release left nostril and exhale slowly to a count of six.
Repeats. Breathe regularly for a few moments, then repeat once.

If you get out of breath when running you are probably not fit, but you may also be breathing wrongly.

there's no easy way

If you find the idea of exercising regularly for the rest of your life rather daunting, remember that there is simply no other way to keep in shape. So long as people are lazy enough to look for easy ways to keep trim, 'miracle' treatments will be invented to fill the bill. Some may help temporarily, others will not help at all—and none can be a substitute for the real thing.

Massage is certainly soothing for tired muscles—but it cannot actually strengthen them. You may find a regular massage does wonders for tension and keeps your skin supple—but it certainly will not tone up flabby thighs or reduce your hip-measurement. This applies to both hand and mechanical massage.

Exercise Machines, such as belts and rollers, will probably improve circulation and have a warming, relaxing effect—but they do not have any miracle inch-whittling effect. The sad fact is that you could use a vibrating body-belt every day for a year and still not lose an inch.

Faradic Massage Machines will improve muscle tone—but the result is only temporary. However, as an incentive at the start of a figure-improving campaign these can be useful—providing that the toned muscles are kept strong with ordinary exercise later on. Started approximately six weeks after childbirth, for example, a course of faradic treatments can dramatically improve stomach muscles, but they will soon sag again once the treatments stop.

Inflatable 'Slimming' Garments will make you hot and uncomfortable but they will not improve your shape. Fluid lost by perspiration is rapidly replaced as soon as you drink something, so even temporary weight-loss would be quickly made up. As for muscle-tone, slimming garments can do nothing for that!

'Slimming' Wraps are one of the newest 'rapid' slimming treatments. They appear to produce a significant inch-loss (although you have to spend an uncomfortable couple of hours wrapped in bandages soaked in a special 'secret' solution) but, again, this is quickly replaced. Most beauticians use this treatment as an incentive only. The real figure-trimming work is done with diet and exercise.

how to use this exercise plan

On the following pages there are exercises to suit everyone, including a planned scheme of exercises which progresses from simple limbering exercises to those suited to the really fit.

Do not be too ambitious

The exercise section has been arranged progressively. First two really easy sections, neither of which is time-consuming—exercises to do in the office or car, and some to do in the bath. The next two sections, yoga and exercises for hands, feet and head will get you warmed up and relaxed before you start your full exercise routine. The hand and feet exercises tone up circulation and help you to avoid painful cramps, while the yoga poses help you to find out what shape you are in.

You must start the exercise course (pages 98-115) right from the beginning and gradually work up to the more difficult exercises as you become proficient. Do not leap straight into the 'Thirty minute a day work-out'—the exercises will be far too difficult, and you could injure yourself. Even if you stay at the very beginning of the course—the limbering-up exercises—for several months, do not worry. It is far better to stick to a regular routine of easy exercises than to tackle a difficult one and then give up.

Choose your moment

Try to set aside a regular time of day for your exercise session—even if it is only 10 minutes before breakfast. Two or three well-chosen exercises will do wonders for problem areas if they are done regularly, but very little if they are taken as an occasional panic measure. You should look forward to your exercises—if you do not then switch to another routine.

Before you start

Remember the following rules:
1. If you want to exercise because of a particular health problem—a slipped disc, for example, or simply to regain strength after an operation—you must consult your doctor first. And you must show him the particular exercises which you propose to do.
2. Always start gently with one or two repetitions of a simple movement. A violent opening exercise will be too much of a shock for your body, and it could be harmful.
3. Never exercise on a full stomach.
4. Watch out for obstacles. None of these exercises take up much space, but before you swing into action it is wise to make sure you will not collide with precious ornaments, doorknobs, fruit-bowls or anything else.

Study the instructions

Read the exercise and breathing instructions carefully before you begin. Try out each movement slowly, studying the illustrations as you work.

Wear something comfortable

Do not try to do exercises in ordinary, work-a-day clothes. Wear shorts, old jeans (no tight waistbands), T-shirt, leotard or stretchy vest and pants or nothing—whatever is most comfortable. It is best not to wear shoes—tights, socks, bare feet or the softest ballet pumps are better as they give your feet freedom of movement.

Enjoy exercise

Exercise can and should be fun. If you regard your daily exercise routine as a necessary chore you may skimp it or, worse still, give up altogether. So, if you think you will find it difficult to set aside time everyday to exercise start by doing the isometric exercises and the bath exercises. When, after this painless introduction, you begin to feel the benefits of regular exercise you will probably feel you want to embark on the more ambitious exercise scheme.

exercise wherever you go, whatever you do

The principle of the isometric exercise is simple: the muscle is contracted through pushing, pressing, pulling or squeezing against an immovable object. This contraction helps to tone and strengthen the muscle—and has the advantage of being easily combined with other physical activities. It is often unobtrusive, too.

So, using this technique, extend your exercise programme to include some useful, effective isometrics that can be done outside the home—in the office, while waiting for a bus or while sitting in your car in a traffic jam.

Saving time

This is one exercise method which should appeal to those people who swear they simply have not got the time to devote to a regular programme. If you practise these movements often enough you find that they become almost automatic, And they take up no time, for you do them while doing something else—answering the telephone, for example.

Aches and pains

Some of the office exercises included in the programme have the added advantage of relaxing and toning tired muscles. So you will find that you feel less fatigued and irritable at the end of a working day.

Unobtrusive exercise

These isometric exercises have been deliberately chosen so that they can be done unobtrusively, at your office desk or during a car journey. Be sensible in your approach—fit the exercises in as and when they seem appropriate. There is no need to stop working while you do them. Finally, remember that while the movements themselves may be unobtrusive you will reveal your secret if you allow the effort to show on your face—and clenched teeth or rolling eyes do not make the exercise easier or more effective and do not tone facial muscles.

The exercises

1. To tone Pectoral muscles
Sit at your desk (or a desk-sized table) with back straight, feet together (in the position described in detail on pages 8-9). Now spread your arms and grip the outside edges of your desk. Squeeze in hard with your hands. Hold for a count of six, then relax.
Breathing. Take a deep breath before starting to squeeze hands, then breathe out slowly as you hold the position.
Repeats. Rest, then repeat 5 times.

2. To tone inside thigh muscles
Sitting comfortably on a straight-backed chair with arms relaxed, grip a waste-paper basket between the inner edges of your feet. Squeeze your feet together as hard as you can. Hold for a count of six, then relax.
Breathing. Breathe regularly throughout the exercise.
Repeats. Repeat 5 times.

1.

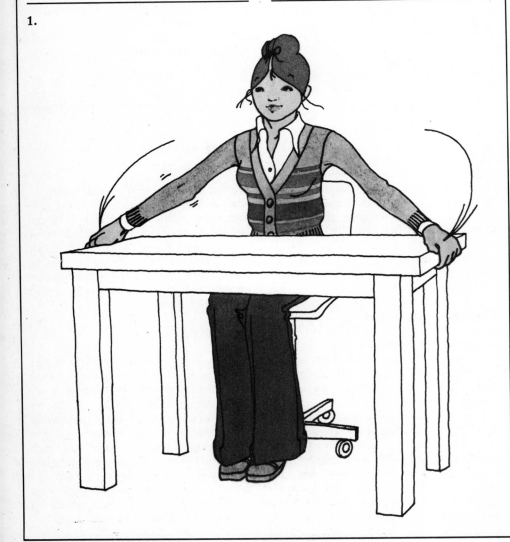

Exercise 2 (right) can be done in the office or the home—all you need is a waste-paper basket.

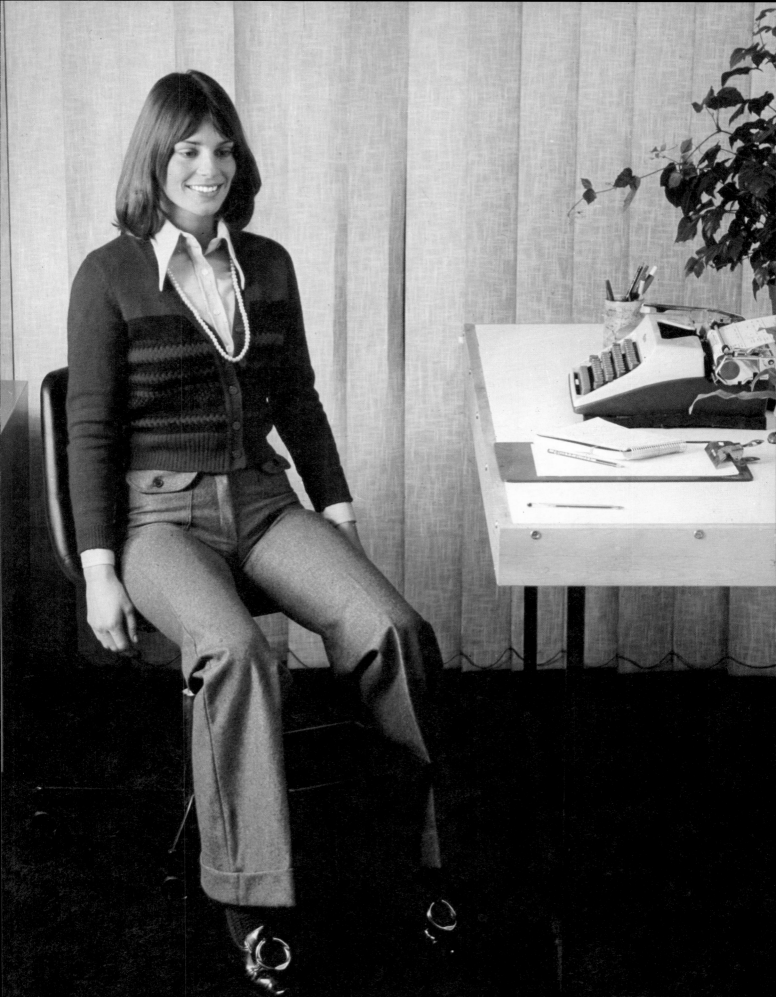

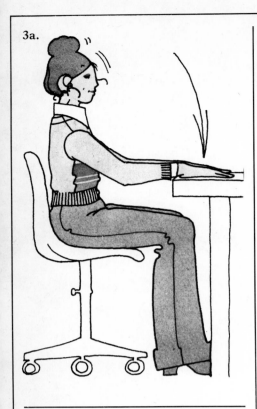

3a.

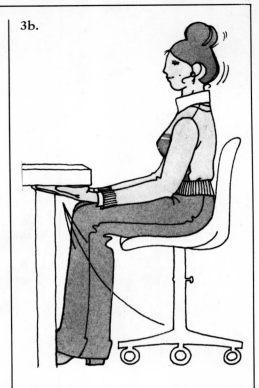

3b.

3. To firm flabby upper arm muscles

a. Sitting at your desk (or desk-sized table) with back straight and feet together, place the palms of your hands flat on the desk-top about one inch apart.

Now press down as hard as you can—almost as though you were trying to force the table into the floor. Hold for a count of six, then relax.

b. Now place the palms of your hands beneath the edge of the desk. Keep your elbows tucked in against your sides and press upwards as hard as you can (if the table is light, weight it down with something heavy). Hold for a count of six, then relax.

Breathing. Breathe in as you start to press your hands up or down, out as you hold the position.

Repeats. Repeat the whole exercise 5 times.

4.

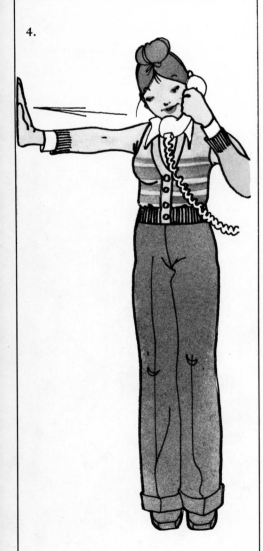

5.

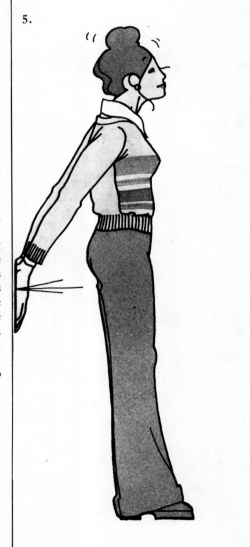

4. To tone arm, shoulder and back muscles

While taking a telephone call, stand at arm's length away from a convenient wall. Hold the receiver to your ear with one hand and push the palm of the other hand hard against the wall. Hold for a count of six, then relax.

Breathing. Breathe regularly throughout the exercise (you will be talking, too).

Repeats. Repeat 5 times, then change hands and repeat a further 5 times.

5. To tone upper arm, shoulder and back muscles

Stand with your back to a tall filing cabinet (or a wall will do) about nine inches away from it. Keeping your legs straight, feet slightly apart and arms straight, reach backwards and press the palms of your hands flat against the filing cabinet. Now push back hard with both hands. Hold for a count of six, then relax.

Breathing. Breathe in as you start to push, out as you hold the position.

Repeats. Repeat 5 times.

6.

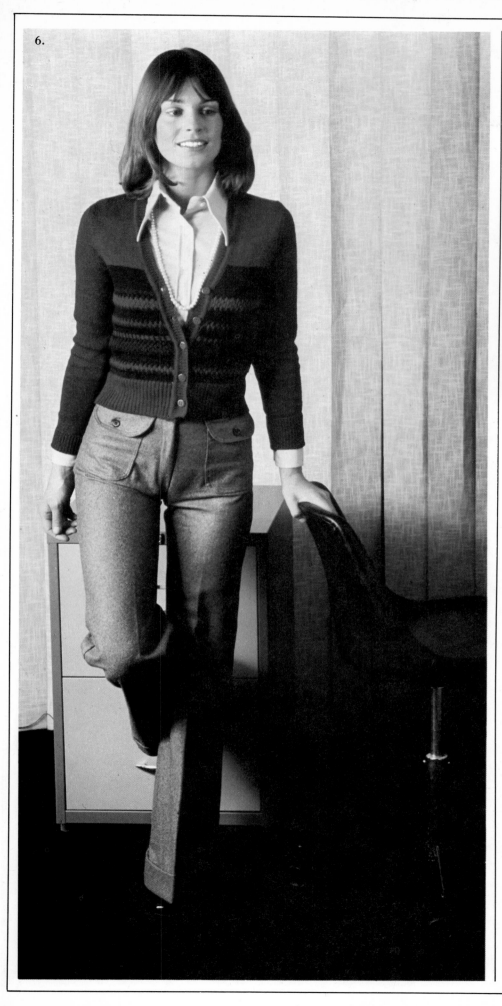

7.

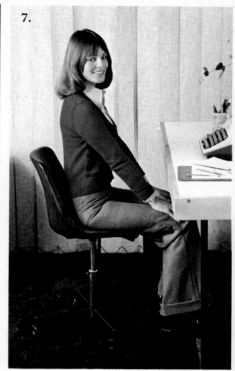

6. To tone the upper leg rear muscles

Stand straight with your back about one foot from a filing cabinet (or chest of drawers). Raise your right foot until it rests under the handle of the second to bottom drawer of the filing cabinet. Rest your left hand on a chair back for balance.

Now press your right heel hard against the drawer handle pulling up against it. (You should feel the back thigh muscles contracting.) Hold for a count of six then relax.

Breathing. Breathe regularly throughout the exercise.

Repeats. Relax and repeat 5 times.

7. To strengthen upper back and stomach muscles

Sit comfortably on a straight-backed chair, feet together, back straight. Now part your knees and place your feet firmly on the floor about one inch apart. Place the palms of your hands flat on your thighs. Keeping your arms straight, press downwards strongly pulling in your stomach muscles at the same time. Hold for a count of six, then relax.

Breathing. Breathe in as you start to press down, and hold the breath as you count six. Breathe out as you relax.

Repeats. Repeat 5 times.

8. To strengthen wrists and forearms

Stand near a bus-stop or any vertical pole and grip the pole with both hands, right hand above the left hand and arms bent. Now move your arms as if to twist the right hand in an anti-clockwise direction and the left hand in a clockwise direction—but resisting the effort as you do so. Hold for a count of six then relax.

Breathing. Breathe regularly throughout the exercise.

Repeats. Repeat 5 times.

8.

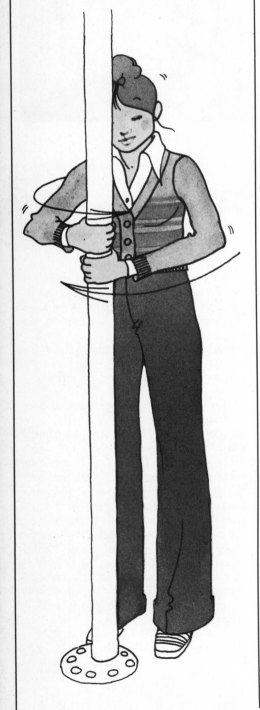

9. To tone arm and Pectoral muscles

While waiting in a traffic jam—but never just while waiting for traffic lights to change—use the time for some simple exercises. Grip the steering wheel at the '9 o'clock' and '3 o'clock' positions, and squeeze it in your hands hard. Hold for as long as possible, then relax.

Breathing. Breathe regularly throughout the exercise.

Repeats. Repeat as often as time allows.

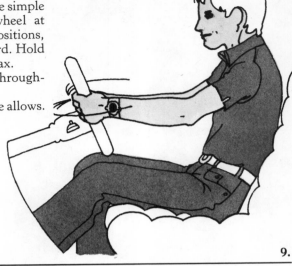

9.

10. To strengthen back muscles

Still sitting in that traffic jam, grip the steering wheel at the position described above. Now straighten your arms and push back as hard as possible against the seat-back behind you. Hold for as long as possible, then relax.

Breathing. Breathe regularly throughout the exercise.

Repeats. Repeat as often as time allows.

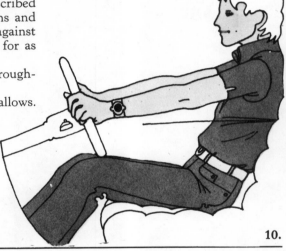

10.

11. To tone thigh muscles

Still while caught in that traffic jam, and holding the steering wheel in the position described above, press your heels back hard against the front of the seat. Hold for as long as possible, then relax.

Breathing. Breathe regularly throughout the exercise.

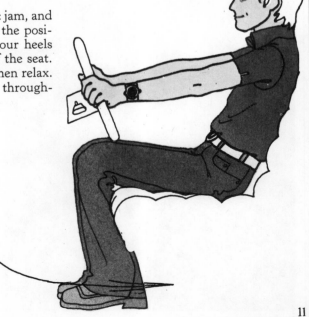

11.

exercises in the bath

Bath-exercising is particularly effective because very little actual muscular fatigue is experienced. The body is independent of gravity and body-weight is reduced to a few pounds. The buoyancy of the water supports the body like a cushion. This makes it an especially good method of exercising for the elderly or those weakened by illness. If you suspect that your bath is too short or too long for you to do all the exercises comfortably try them out with no water in the bath. If your bath is too long it is better to find out beforehand that your head would be under water if you laid back rather than to attempt it in a full bath and half-drown yourself!

Remember, too, to wear a bath-cap to protect your hair if you have had it set.

Your exercise bath

Take your bath at least 2 hours after your last meal and make sure that the water-level is such that, when you lie back, it comes up to your neck. The water temperature is up to you—make sure you are comfortable and warm throughout the session. Perform the various exercises smoothly—waves will certainly appear, but they should not be boisterous enough to flood the bathroom. Keep breathing smooth and even, inhaling and exhaling through the nose.

The exercises

1. To strengthen stomach, thighs and lower back muscles
Lie back in the bath with your arms by your side, feet together and head resting comfortably on the end of the bath. (A bath pillow is useful here.)
Now slowly raise your arms to the horizontal position, bending knees and lifting feet at the same time. Point your toes and hold the position for a count of six. Lower feet and arms slowly.
Breathing. Breathe out as you raise arms and knees, in as you lower them.
Repeats. Repeat 10 times.

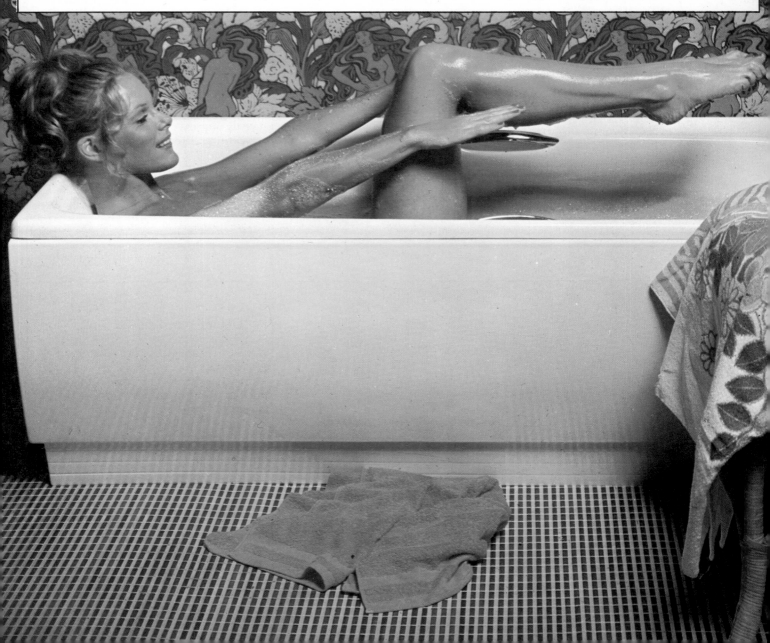

2.

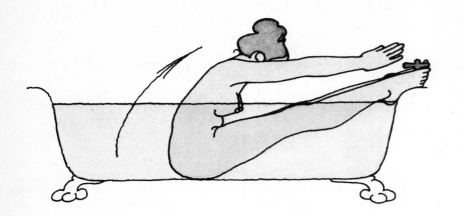

2. To strengthen stomach muscles and tone legs, hips, back, shoulders and arms

Lie back in the bath with your legs extended and your toes wedged under the taps, arms by your sides.

Now sit up slowly and carry on the movement as if to touch your knees with your face, stretching out your arms to touch your toes at the same time. Hold for a count of ten then slowly lie back again.

Breathing. Breathe out as you stretch forward, in as you lean back.

Repeats. Repeat 10 times.

3.

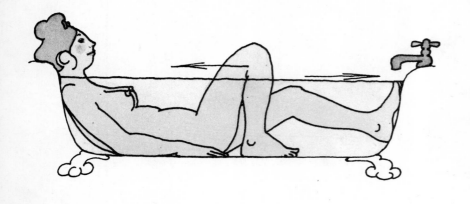

3. To strengthen stomach, buttocks and thighs

Lie back in the bath with your hands resting on the bottom.

Now draw your right heel back along the bottom of the bath towards your right buttock. Then straighten the leg, and start drawing up the left heel at the same time. Keep the movement going evenly and rhythmically.

Breathing. Breathe in as you bend your knee, out as you straighten your leg.

Repeats. 10 with each leg, then 10 drawing up both legs together.

4.

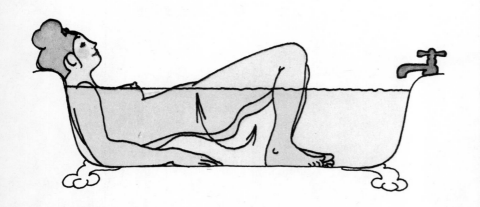

4. To tone waistline and hips

Lie back in the bath, resting on your forearms and elbows at each side of your body.

Now slide back your feet so that they are flat on the bottom of the bath. Slowly raise your hips and buttocks off the bottom of the bath, keeping your body in a straight line and taking the strain, if any, on your arms and elbows. (You will notice that this is far easier than it sounds because of the buoyancy of the bath water.) When hips are raised, swing them gently and evenly from side to side.

Breathing. Breathe regularly throughout the exercise.

Repeats. Swing 10 times to each side.

5. To tone thighs, buttocks, stomach, arms, shoulders and the Pectoral muscles

Lie back in the bath with your feet together floating just on top of the surface of the water.

Now stretch out your arms along your sides with your palms resting on the surface of the water. (Make sure your head is comfortably supported by the end of the bath.) Then press your feet and hands towards the bottom of the bath at the same time, keeping them stiff and making sure you feel the resistance of the water. Relax back to starting position.

Breathing. Breathe out as you press down feet and hands, in as you relax.

Repeats. Repeat the whole exercise 10 times, resting between each one for a count of four.

5.

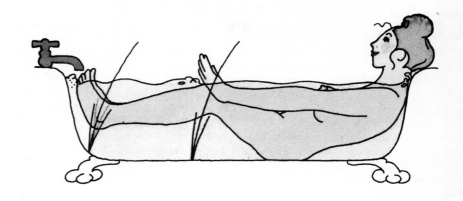

6. To trim the waistline

Sit up in the bath, resting your feet comfortably on the bottom, with your legs slightly apart.

Now clasp your hands behind your head making sure that your back is straight and head held high. Twist your trunk slowly to the right—going as far as is comfortably possible. Hold for a count of three, then return to starting position and relax for a count of three. Then twist to the left, hold for a count of three and return to starting position.

Breathing. Breathe out as you twist, in as you come back to starting position.

Repeats. Repeat the whole exercise 10 times.

6.

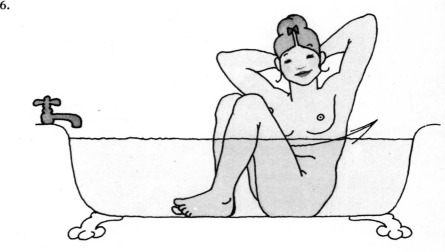

7. To strengthen stomach muscles

Lie back comfortably in the bath, your feet resting on the bottom and your hands floating by your sides.

Now pull in your stomach muscles towards the base of your spine. Hold for a count of three then release and rest for a count of three.

Breathing. Breathe out deeply before you pull in stomach muscles, breathe in as you release.

Repeats. Repeat 5 times, resting in between.

7.

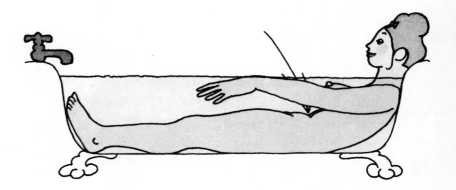

exercises for relaxation—yoga

True relaxation is an art in itself, and can be achieved by exercise—particularly yoga. If that sounds contradictory, remember that for 3,000 years complete physical and mental relaxation has been taught by the Yogis of India who use controlled exercise as an important part of their teaching. This ancient technique has an important part to play in any modern exercise programme—particularly when the programme is directed at people who have not exercised regularly for many years. *Hatha-yoga* is made up of a series of movements which are slow and rigorously controlled. These movements are called *Asanas* and are made up of three distinct phases: first, the posture is assumed, slowly and surely, making the muscles work in a progressive fashion; second, the posture is held for several seconds (this is known as the 'static' phase and it should be a period of intense concentration and regular breathing); finally, there is the slow return to the original position from the 'static' phase. This must be achieved with economy of movement and, again, great muscular control. The completion of each *Asana* is followed by total relaxation, lying flat on your back.

What does this slow, controlled form of exercise achieve? Firstly, each *Asana* makes several sets of muscles work hard and also helps to make the joints more supple. Then, there are also the internal effects. Yoga helps to stimulate the intestines and the liver and helps to regulate the elimination of waste products. It is also said to regulate the metabolism (many slimmers have found it a tremendous help when accompanied by a low-calorie diet) and to relieve rheumatism and arthritis. Certainly, the regular practice of yoga *Asanas* has a calming effect on the mind and produces suppleness in the body. It also helps to improve the circulation and develop concentration.

All in the mind

Because it is impossible to tackle a yoga programme when you are rushed or trying to think of something else, the technique literally forces you to relax. Your thoughts are turned away from outside influences and inwards on your body. Each pose demands total concentration, and after an average 15-minute session the feeling of refreshment and tranquillity which flows over you is as good as that which follows a night's sleep. You are relaxed, but at the same time you are mentally alert and physically in top form.

Prepare yourself

You cannot just throw yourself into a yoga session; the conditions have to be right. You need:

Silence. Yoga *Asanas* must be performed in an atmosphere of peace, with no groups of giggling beginners, blaring music or ringing telephones to disturb your concentration.

Comfortable clothing. Do not try to perform yoga poses in tight clothing.

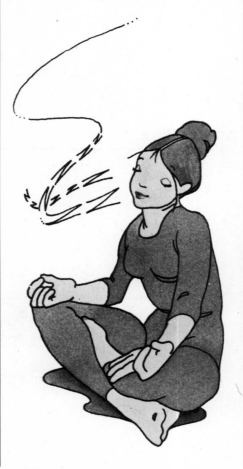

The best thing to wear is a leotard or sweater and tights, or nothing.

A rug or carpet. Yoga poses are uncomfortable if you do them on a bare floor. Use a large rug or blanket spread on a carpet.

Timing

The best time of day for yoga is early morning, as it does seem to set you up for the day. However, at any time of particular tension or strain, a short yoga session can help you to unwind and recoup your energies.

Aims

Each of the simple yoga *Asanas* shown on the next four pages should be performed with economy of movement—in the first phase no wavering in the air or wobbling. And when the pose is successfully achieved, try to release all the muscles not directly involved in the action. Once you can hold the pose comfortably for some time you will know that your posture is good. During the rest phase after each pose you should concentrate on regular, deep breathing. Never force yourself into a pose which is uncomfortable or a strain. Just go as far as you can, rest and try again next time. As with any system of exercise, the more you practise, the more you will be able to achieve, and the more you will benefit. However, do not spend longer than 20 minutes or so a day doing yoga.

How yoga fits into this programme

Yoga has been introduced at this point for several reasons.

First, it is a good idea to concentrate on complete relaxation and to take stock of one's physical condition. Yoga is the perfect way to awareness of the possibilities, and limitations, of one's own body. Each pose or *Asana* tests a certain set of muscles and by regular practice you will be able to find out where any weaknesses lie.

Second, yoga is ideal for a warming-up period before beginning more strenuous movement because it exercises your body gently, without excessive exertion or strain and with the minimum of nervous fatigue. And it is a good idea to finish any period of strenuous exercise with the pose for relaxation.

When doing your yoga exercises wear something comfortable and concentrate on graceful, fluid movements.

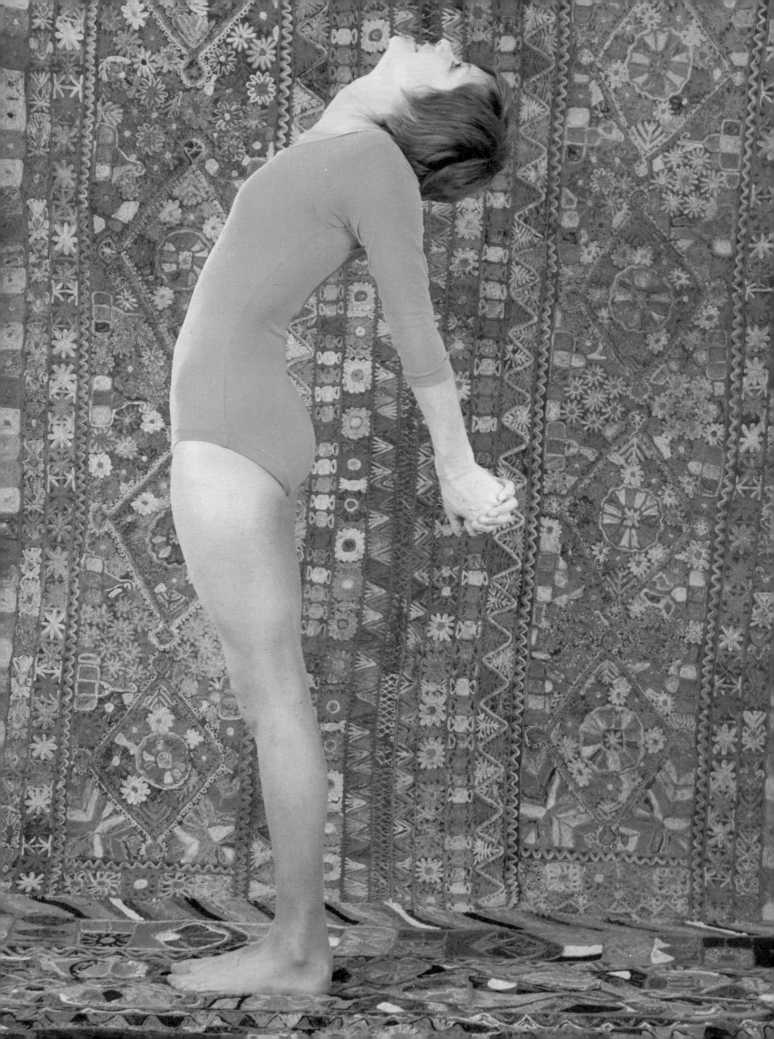

The exercises

1. To relieve tension from back and spine

Lie on your stomach, legs straight, feet together, arms resting lightly by your sides. Place your left cheek on the floor. Relax completely.

Now turn your head and rest your forehead on the floor. Bring your hands underneath your shoulders, fingers touching. Slowly push your hands against the floor and raise your trunk, tilting your head back as you do so, until your arms are straight and your spine is curving backwards.

Hold this position for a count of ten, then slowly return to the starting position and relax.

Breathing. Breathe out as you start the exercise, in as you raise trunk.

Repeats. Relax and repeat once.

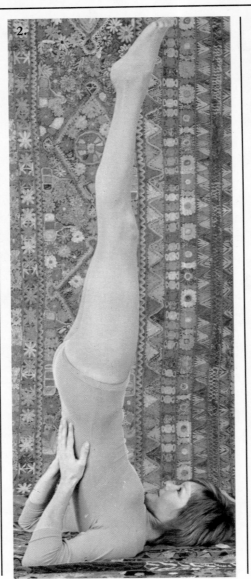

2. To improve circulation

Lie on your back, with your feet together, legs straight, arms by your sides. Relax completely.

Now slowly raise both legs to the vertical position, making sure they are straight. (You will find this easier to do if at the same time you push down with the palms of your hands on the floor.) Hold for a count of five.

Now press down on the floor again and raise the lower half of your body. Place your hands under your hips to prop yourself up. Straighten legs and extend your whole body up on your shoulders as near as possible to a vertical position (this is often called a shoulder-stand), pointing your toes as you do so. Hold this position for as long as is comfortably possible, then lower your body very gently to first position and relax.

Breathing. Breathe in as you start the exercise, out as you raise your legs.

Repeats. Relax and repeat once.

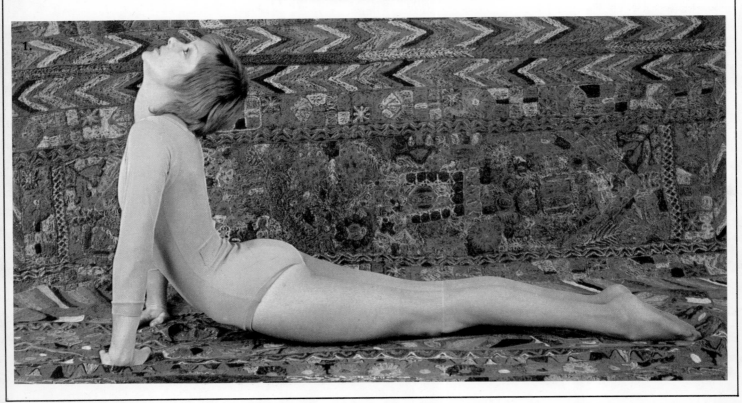

3. To improve posture, strengthen and firm bustline

a. Stand straight, feet together, spine relaxed, arms at your sides.
Now slowly bring your arms up and touch your chest with your hands, palms outwards. Slowly straighten your arms, stretching your elbows as you do so.

b. Now bring your arms behind you at shoulder level, then lower them slightly and clasp your fingers behind you.

c. Slowly bend backwards (just a few inches) and look upwards. Hold for a count of ten.

d. Now bend forward, bringing your arms high over your back (fingers must still be clasped). Hold for a count of 20. Straighten to upright position, unclasp hands and relax.

Breathing. Breathe out as you straighten your arms, in as you bring them behind you, out as you clasp fingers, in as you bend backwards. Breathe regularly as you hold first position, breathe out as you bend forward, in as you straighten up.

Repeats. Relax and repeat once.

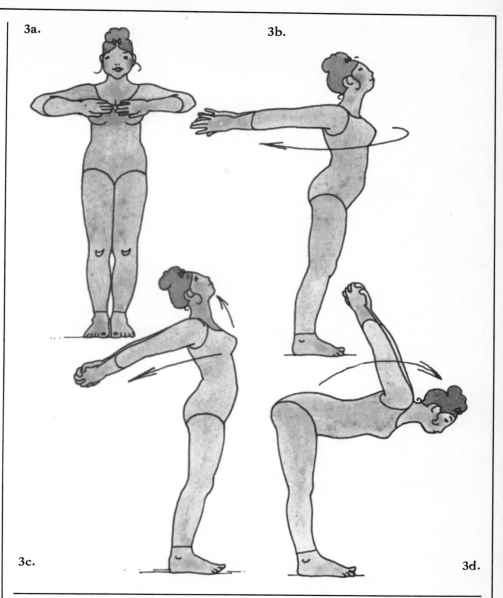

3a.

3b.

3c.

3d.

4. To make back and spine stronger and more flexible

a. Sit on the floor, feet together, back straight, hands resting lightly on your thighs with elbows bent.
Now raise your arms slowly to shoulder level, then overhead. Bend backwards several inches.

b. Keeping your arms outstretched, bend slowly forwards to hold knees securely. Bend your elbows and draw your whole trunk downwards (forehead aiming at your knees) as far as possible. (Knees and legs must remain straight throughout.) Hold the position for a count of 20 then straighten up and slide your hands back up to your thighs. Relax.

Breathing. Breathe in as you raise your hands, out as you bend forward, regularly as you hold position, in again as you straighten up.

Repeat. Relax and repeat once.

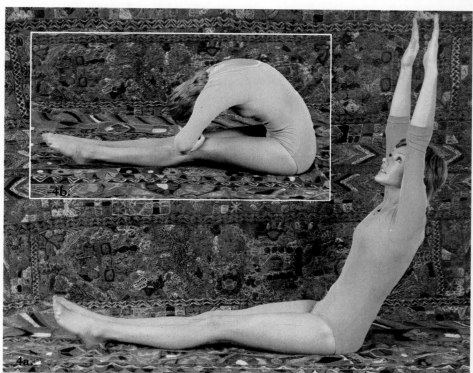

4b.

4a.

5b.

5c.

5d.

5. To loosen hip and shoulder joints
a. Lie on your back, feet together, legs straight, arms by your sides.
b. Now bend your knees, part them and press the soles of your feet together. Stretch your arms over your head and let them rest, palms upward, on the floor behind you.
c. Next, keeping your knees parted and legs bent, cross one foot over the other.
d. Then cross your arms behind your head. Hold this position for a count of 20 then straighten your arms and legs and relax.
Breathing. Breathe regularly throughout the exercise.
Repeats. Relax and repeat once.

6. To make the spine, hip and knee joints flexible and develop concentration
a. Lie on the floor in the position held in the last exercise.
b. Now sit up slowly, using your hands to help you, but keeping your feet in the 'crossed-over' position. Straighten your back and let your arms fall loosely to your sides.
c. Now clasp your hands behind your back and lean forward slowly, keeping your arms flexible, and allow your head to touch the floor. Hold the position for a count of ten then raise your body and relax.
Breathing. Breathe in the sitting position, out as you lean forward. Breathe regularly as you hold the position, then breathe in as you straighten up.
Repeats. Relax and repeat once.

7. To relax the body completely
a. Lie on the floor, feet together, and place the fingertips of both hands on the top of your abdomen. Close your eyes. Breathe slowly and quietly for several minutes, allowing all muscles to relax. Inhale slowly, hold your breath and move your fingertips to rest lightly on your forehead.
b. Exhale slowly. Transfer fingertips to abdomen, and repeat whole exercise.
Breathing. As given in the exercise instructions. It is important to concentrate completely on your breathing—and nothing else.
Repeats. Repeat 7 times. Relax, arms by your sides, breathing normally.

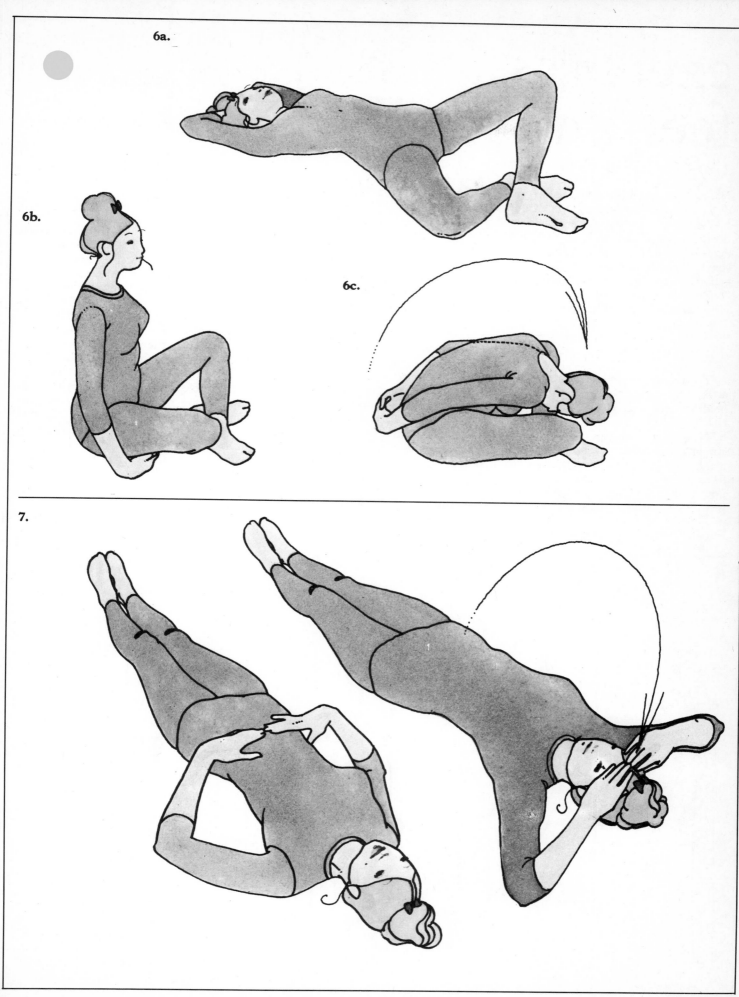

6a.

6b.

6c.

7.

exercises for hands, feet and head

Hands and feet—the extremities—are often the most neglected parts of our bodies, and yet they are expected to do the most work. Walking does not exercise all the muscles of the feet—some get neglected—and everyday hand activities (writing, typing, gardening, cooking etc.) do not give fingers and wrists all the exercise they need.

If you are prone to cramp, aching feet, stiff finger joints or chilblains you have an extra reason for making sure all the muscles in those important extremities are exercised regularly and circulation is kept pepped up.

These exercises are simple to do. Use them as a preliminary to your main exercise session and you will find that your feet and hands will be more supple for the movements in the general body exercises. Also try them when you have a spare moment—if your fingers get tired while typing or writing, or if your toes feel cold or numb while you are waiting for the bed to warm up. Night cramp sufferers should do the toes, feet and ankle exercises for a few minutes before getting into bed. (It is better to keep your own circulation going than rely on artificial aids.)

The exercises

1. To strengthen feet and ankles
a. Sit on a chair, back straight, hands holding lightly on to the sides of the chair-seat.
b. Now raise your legs, keeping them straight, to a position about one inch off the floor. Point your toes hard downwards and then pull your feet upwards, curling your toes up towards you. Repeat several times.
c. Now open your legs so that your feet are about six inches apart and rotate feet outwards and inwards alternately.
Breathing. Breathe regularly throughout the exercise.
Repeats. Repeat the movements alternately for about 3 minutes.

2. To strengthen feet and toes
Stand straight, with your hands by your sides and your feet together.
Now raise yourself on tiptoe. Hold for a count of six, then lower.
Breathing. Breathe regularly throughout the exercise.
Repeats. Repeat 5 times.

3. To strengthen wrists and fingers
Raise hands to ear level, about six inches away from your face. Now, using the whole hand, make flowing movements from the wrist, carrying the movement all through the hand to the tips of your fingers—almost as if you were an Eastern dancer.
Breathing. Breathe regularly throughout the exercise.
Repeats. Repeat movement for about 1 minute.

Exercise 3., see facing page.

1b.

1c.

2.

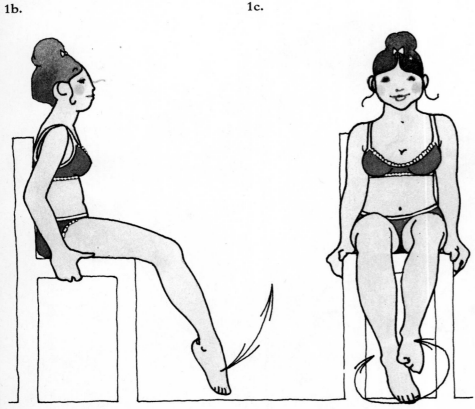

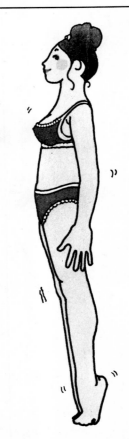

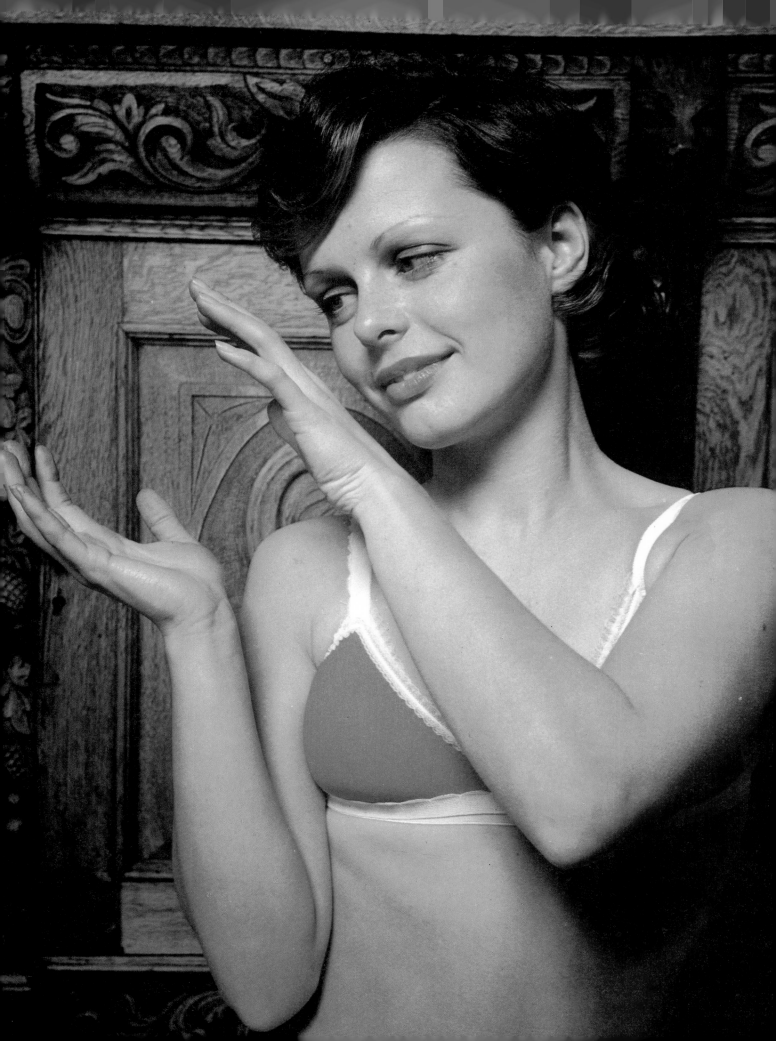

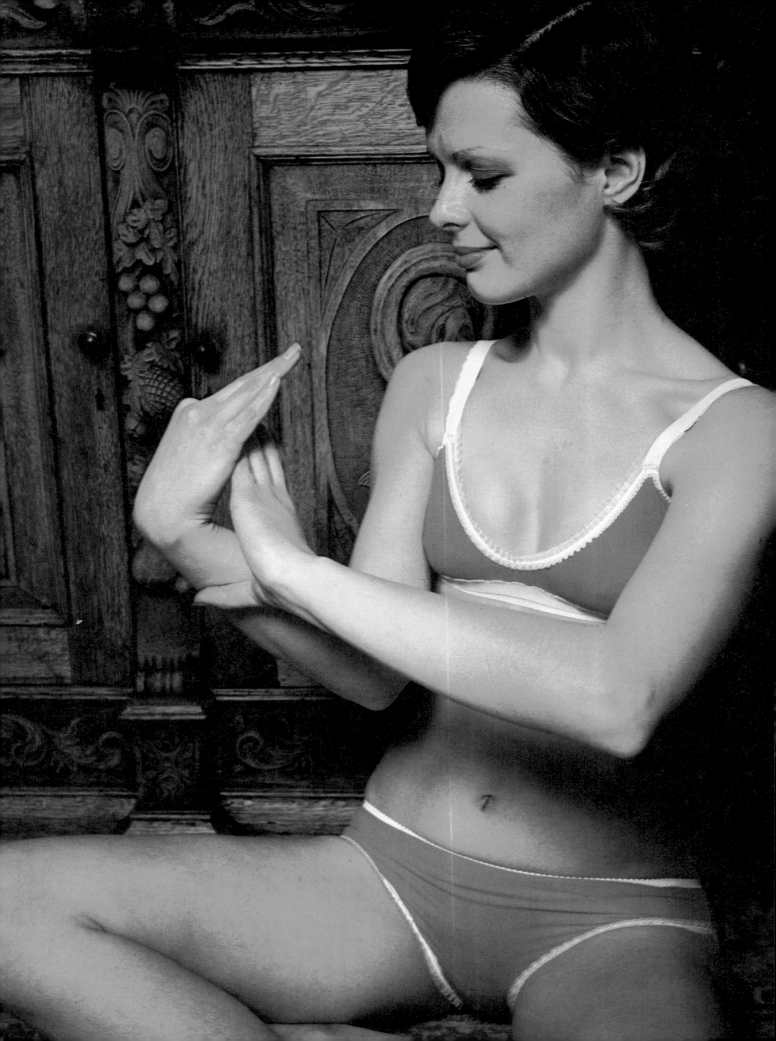

4. To strengthen hands and wrists

a. Sit down on the floor, spread out your fingers on the floor and press down and relax rhythmically for a few seconds.
b. Now, holding your hand in the air, hold your right wrist with the four fingers of your left hand. Bend your wrist forward and pull each finger of your right hand in towards the palm of your right hand with the thumb of your left hand. Repeat with whole hand twice, then repeat with other hand.
c. Now clench your fists and hold your hands in front of your chest. Spread your fingers and fling your hands outwards five times.
d. Finally, let your hands hang limply and shake them rapidly in circular movements.
Breathing. Breathe regularly throughout the exercises.
Repeats. Repeat all the movements consecutively for about 5 minutes.

5. To tone face and neck muscles

With your mouth closed and teeth comfortably together, pull the corners of the mouth downwards and outwards. Hold for a count of six, then relax.
Breathing. Breathe regularly throughout the exercise.
Repeats. Repeat 5 times. (And do this exercise in front of a mirror, if possible.)

6. To tone jaw muscles

Open your mouth and try to touch the tip of your nose with your tongue. Hold for a count of three, then relax.
Breathing. Breathe regularly throughout the exercise.
Repeats. Repeat 5 times.

7. To relax and strengthen eye muscles

a. Sit straight, head and chin level and look straight ahead. Without moving your head, roll your eyes in a clockwise position six times, then six times in an anti-clockwise direction.
b. Now focus your gaze alternately on an object on the other side of the room and on one nearby.
c. Now look up, down, and from side to side—still without moving your head.
Breathing. Breathe regularly throughout the exercise.
Repeats. Repeat each movement consecutively for about five minutes.

Exercise 4b., see facing page.

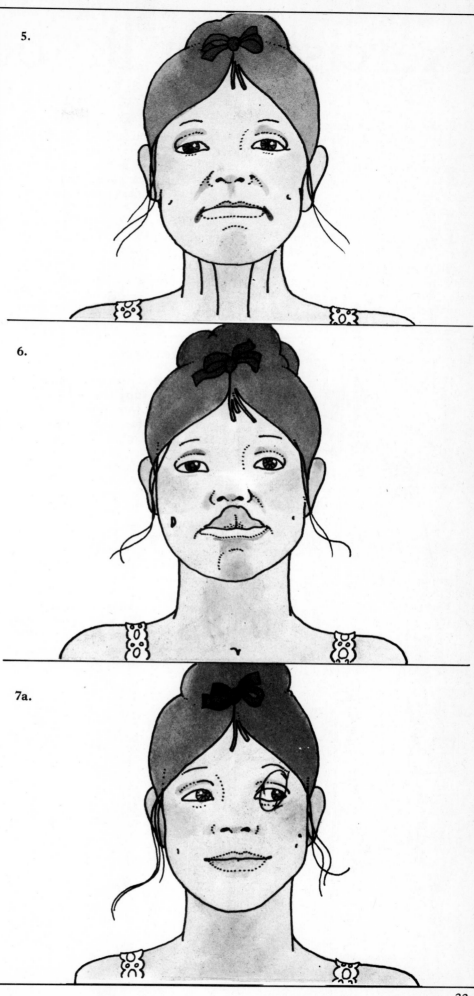

5.

6.

7a.

33

exercises for limbering up

The exercises in this section have been especially devised to help you get into shape gently. None of them is too strenuous or exhausting—so if you are just beginning to exercise you will find that a daily session of these limbering-up exercises will prepare you to move on to the rest of the programme.

Even if you feel that you are fairly fit, it is vital to start with these exercises. Tackling one of the tough sessions in the 'Thirty minutes' a day work-out', pages 109-115, before your body is really supple could mean trouble. This is the stage where you prepare your body for more difficult things—and this is the stage where you should watch your reaction to specific movements very carefully. If you feel any sharp pains when tackling one of the exercises stop and rest. If the pain persists then drop the exercise and consult your doctor. You will certainly feel stiff after a 20-minute limbering-up session, but none of the movements should be painful.

This section is useful to precede any extra physical effort which you may have to make—moving a lot of furniture around, or tackling a strenuous garden job like digging or chopping down trees.

The exercises

1. To improve posture, relax spine and increase suppleness
Stand straight with your back against a wall. Your feet should be a little apart, heels about four inches away from the wall, arms by your sides.

Lean forward from the waist, head hanging down. Now uncurl slowly, so that you feel every knob of your spine against the wall, ending with your head back against it. You should just be able to get your hand between the small of your back and the wall—every other part of your back should be touching the wall.

Breathing. Breathe out as you lean forward, take a slow breath in as you 'uncurl'.

Repeats. Relax for a count of three, then repeat 5 times.

If you are a keen sportsman or sportswoman practise these exercises before you start your summer season of cricket, baseball or tennis. They will prevent those 'first-game twinges' and help you get into top form quickly. Use them, too, as a pre-holiday tonic. Do them for about one week before you travel to the sun. Swimming, walking and even lazing on the beach will then seem more natural and more relaxing—and you will look in better shape, too, because even a week of exercise will improve your posture by making you more aware of your body.

2. To tone back, stomach, thigh and calf muscles
Stand, right foot a little in front of left foot, hands on your hips. Now, keeping your head up, lean slowly forward without raising your heels from the floor, and keeping your back and legs straight throughout. Hold, then straighten up slowly.

It is a good idea to try this exercise sideways-on to a mirror to check your posture as you go.

Breathing. Breathe in when you start the exercise—out as you lean forward.

Repeats. Repeat 4 times, change feet, and repeat a further 4 times.

After just a week of gentle limbering exercises you will feel the benefit of improved posture and (right) increased suppleness in your back.

1.

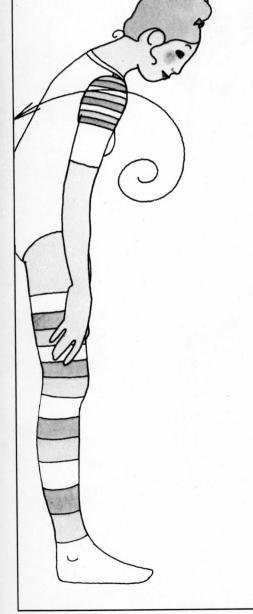

2.

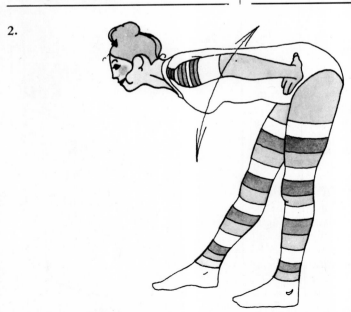

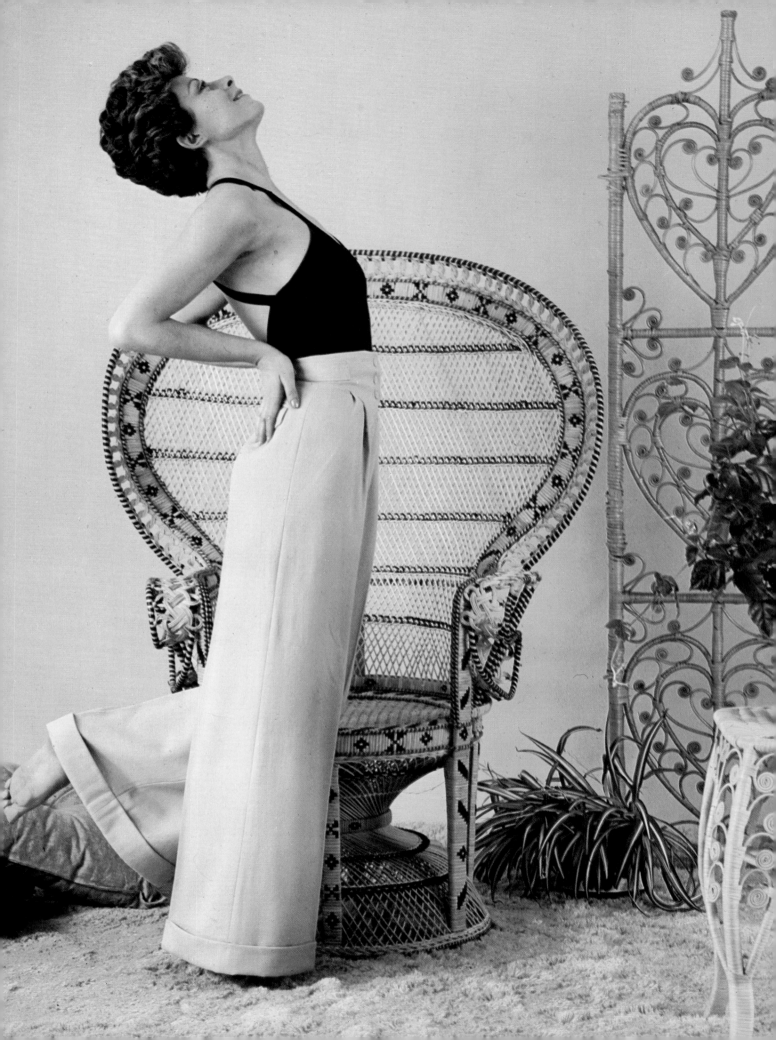

3. To tone back, arms and shoulder muscles, improve posture and relieve tension

a. Stand with feet apart, head hanging down, shoulders relaxed forward with hands hanging forward and backs of hands touching.

b. Now, bring your trunk slowly upwards.

c. Arch your back and bring your arms slowly up and back at the same time, turning palms outwards. Try to make the backs of your hands touch behind you.

Breathing. Breathe out as you hang forwards, in as you bring your trunk up.

Repeats. Repeat the whole exercise 5 times.

3a.

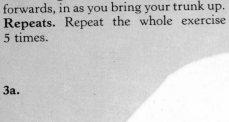

3b.
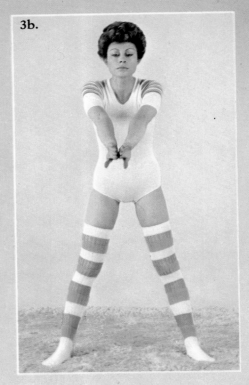

3c.
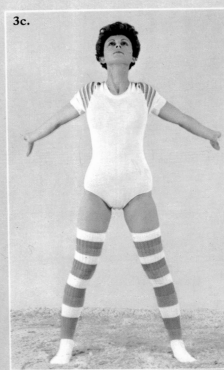

4. To loosen arm, back, shoulder and waist muscles

a. Stand with feet wide apart, head up. Now reach up and 'grab air' with alternate hands, stretching the sides of your body (from hipline upwards) as much as possible. (The movement is very similar to that of climbing a rope.)

b. Next, keeping your feet firmly in position, 'grab air' to the side of your body—stretching first your left hand, then your right hand. Stretch sideways as far as you can—moving from the waistline only.

Breathing. Breathe regularly throughout the exercise.

Repeats. Repeat 10 times 'grabbing air' upwards, then a further 10 times to each side of the body.

5. To loosen hips and lower back, tone calf and thigh muscles

Stand a few feet away from a fairly low chair and, keeping your legs straight, place your left heel on the chair. Grasp your left leg with both hands just above the knee and lean forward slowly, keeping your back straight, your legs straight and your right heel on the ground. You should feel a 'pull' behind your left knee.

Breathing. Breathe regularly throughout the exercise.

Repeats. Repeat 5 times, then a further 5 times with the other leg.

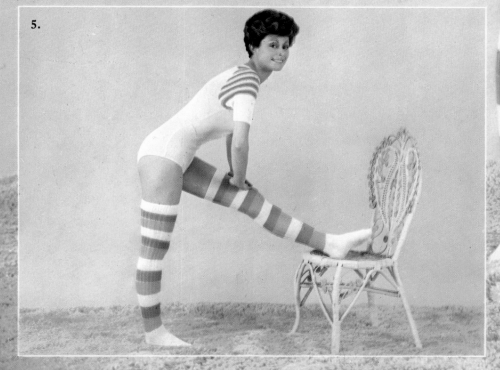

5.

6.

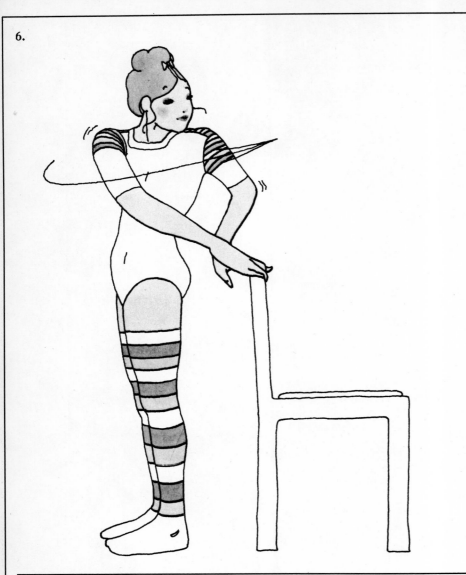

6. To trim waist and trunk muscles

Still using the chair, stand with your back to its back—about arm's distance away. Now keeping feet slightly apart and firmly on the ground, rotate your trunk to grab the back of the chair with both hands, first twisting to the right and then to the left. Your hips should be motionless throughout.

Breathing. Breathe regularly throughout the exercise.

Repeats. Repeat the whole exercise 5 times.

7. To slim thigh muscles and loosen hip joints

a. Still using the chair, stand sideways on to its back—comfortable arm's distance away. Lightly hold the chair-back for balance. Now, with knee slightly bent, swing your outside leg forwards and backwards in an arc of about 45 degrees. Straighten leg and repeat.

Turn around and repeat with the other leg.

b. Now turn to face the chair and swing your left leg across the body and out to the side.

Repeat with the right leg.

Breathing. Breathe in when your leg swings backwards, out when it comes forwards—in when it goes out to the side, out as it goes across your body.

Repeats. Repeat 10-20 times with leg in each position—sideways on and facing the chair-back.

7a.
7b.

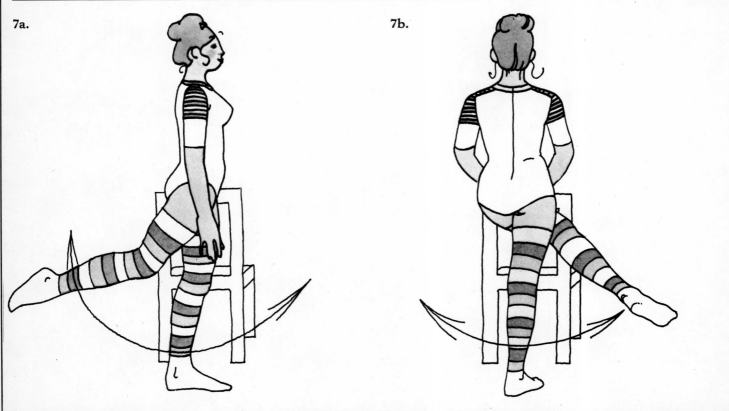

8. To tone Pectoral muscles and loosen shoulder joints

Stand, feet slightly apart, and swing arms backwards in big circles. Use arms singly and then together.

Breathing. Breathe in as you swing arms up, out as you swing them down.

Repeats. Repeat rhythmically for about 30 seconds.

9. To tone neck muscles and relieve tension

a. Kneel on all fours, looking straight ahead and keeping your back straight. Make sure the back of your head is in line with your spine. Turn your head to look over your left shoulder, then your right.

b. Then make a circular movement with your head.

c. Finally, stretch your neck to look up, then down.

Breathing. Breathe regularly throughout the exercise.

Repeats. Repeat each complete movement 10 times.

10. To loosen hips and lower back muscles

Stand, feet slightly apart, hands on hips, stomach tucked in. Now rotate your pelvis, first clockwise then anti-clockwise.

Breathing. Breathe regularly throughout the exercise.

Repeats. Repeat 20 times, rotating pelvis clockwise, then a further 20 times rotating pelvis anti-clockwise.

8.

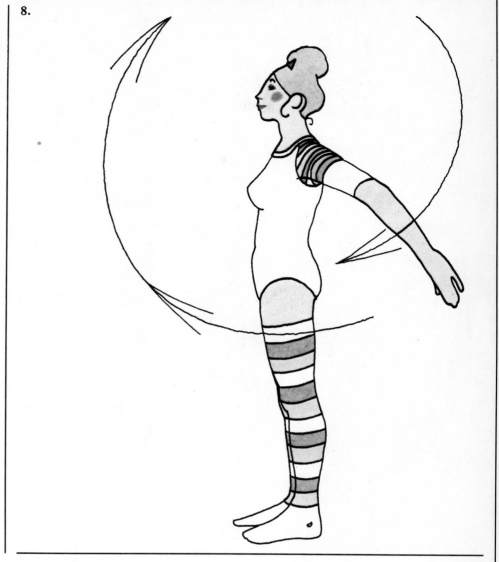

10.

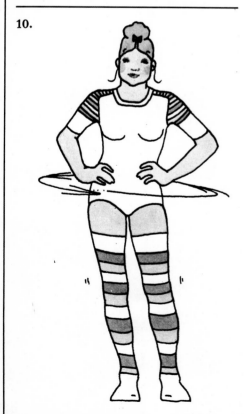

9c.

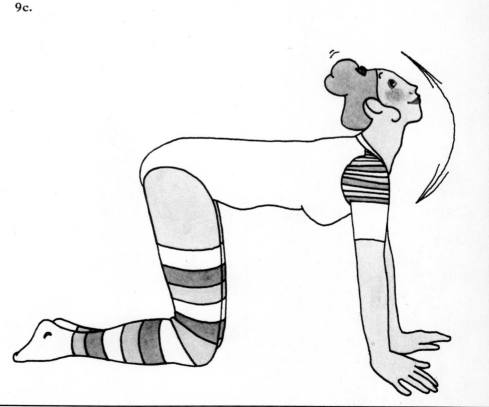

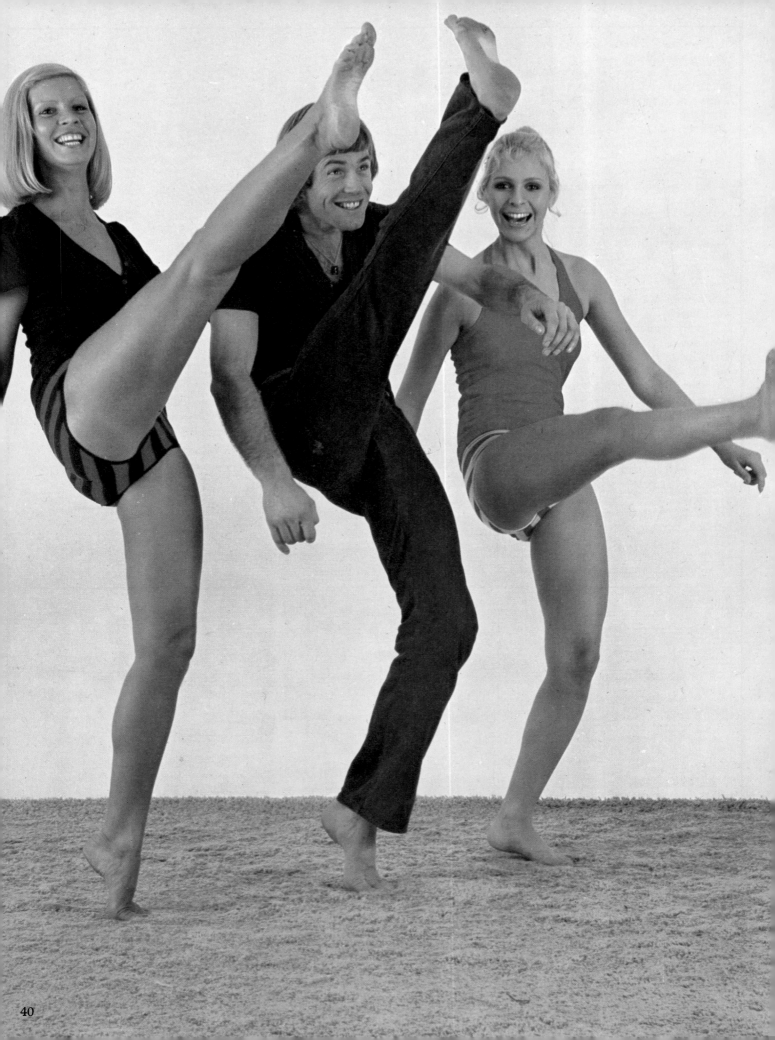

exercises for the fit and lively

After you have warmed up with the limbering-up exercises, and find you can do them easily, it is time to increase the pace a little. This section is fun practised in a group, with a friend or even with young children. In fact, for some of the exercises you must have a partner. And some toe-tapping music will make certain that you keep up the strong rhythm which is an important part of some of the movements.

Put all your energy into this section and really enjoy yourself. If possible, try the exercises out of doors—on the beach, for example. The fresh air will help to improve breathing and circulation.

Try the whole routine at least twice a week. Keep up the pace for about 40 minutes—with a rest halfway through. But do not sit slumped in a chair at rest-time—instead, lie down on the floor in the yoga pose for relaxation—exercise No. 7, page 93.

On the other days of the week do a few exercises to keep yourself in practice—Nos. 6, 8 and 10 if you are alone; 3, 5 and 9 with a partner.

The exercises

1. To tone thigh and stomach muscles and slim buttocks

a. Sit on the floor, with your back straight and head up. Now bend your knees, place the soles of your feet together and pull your feet in close to your body with your hand. Hold your feet with your hands, press your elbows into your knees and use your elbows to push your knees down towards the floor.

b. Now, straighten your arms and, still holding your feet, 'roll' on your bottom from side to side.

Breathing. Breathe regularly throughout the exercise.

Repeats. Repeat each of the two parts for about 30 seconds.

2. To tone stomach, hips and thigh muscles

a. Lie on your back, arms out sideways at shoulder level, feet together. Now slowly bend your knees and bring them up to your stomach, keeping your bottom and shoulders firmly on the floor.

b. Slowly roll both your legs over to the right side—still keeping your bottom as far as possible firmly on the floor—so that your knees touch the floor.

c. Return to knees-on-stomach position and stretch out legs slowly down towards the floor—but keeping them about two inches above floor level.

Breathing. Breathe out as you roll your legs over to the side, in as you return them to knees-on-stomach position.

Repeats. Repeat the whole movement, rolling legs over to the left side, then repeat the whole exercise 10 times.

Bring energy and enthusiasm to your exercise session, particularly to exercises such as 7 (far left). Practise in a group if you can—it does not matter if some members of the group are not as good as others.

1a.

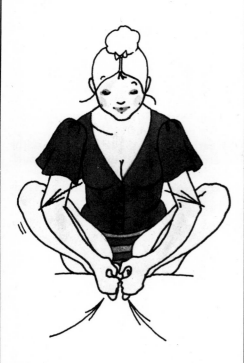

1b.

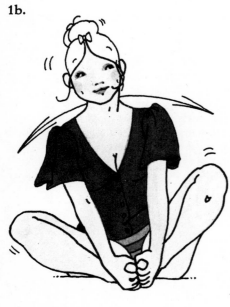

2a.

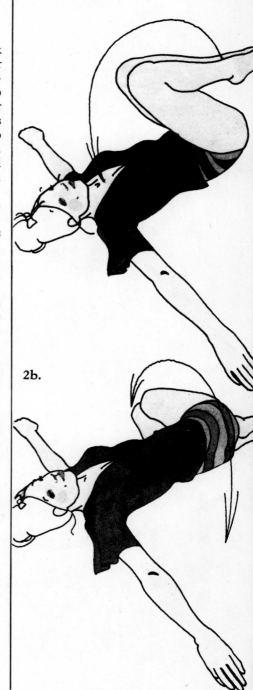

2b.

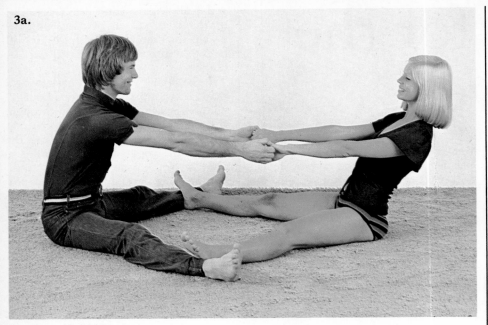

3a.

3. To firm waist, stomach and hips

With a partner, sit on the floor facing each other with legs wide apart. Now brace your feet firmly against your partner's. (If you have shorter legs than your partner, you should tuck your feet inside your partner's for even balance.) Now hold hands:

a. 'See-saw' going alternately backwards and forwards as far as possible and keeping your backs straight throughout.

Breathing. Partner moving backwards breathes in, partner moving forwards breathes out.

Repeats. Repeat the whole movement 10 times.

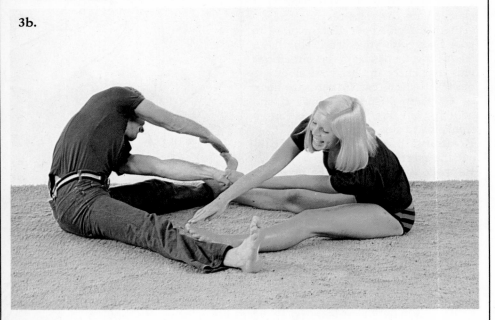

3b.

b. With feet and legs in the same position, grasp your partner's right hand with your right hand. Now, both swing over with your left hands to touch your right toes.

Breathing. Breathe in as you start the exercise, out as you swing over to touch toes.

Repeats. Repeat 10 times, change hands and repeat a further 10 times.

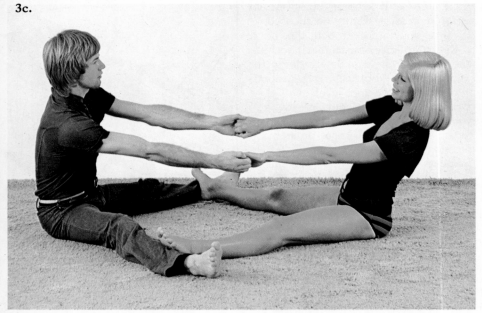

3c.

c. Holding both hands again, alternately lean forward, to the side and backwards, making a large circular movement. Do this first clockwise (first leaning to the right) then anti-clockwise (first leaning to the left).

Breathing. Breathe out as you lean forwards, in as you move round.

Repeats. Repeat whole circle clockwise 5 times, then anti-clockwise 5 times.

4. To firm waist and trunk

(Exercise **a** also slims the thighs.)

With a partner, stand arm's distance apart, facing each other with feet slightly apart. Now hold hands:

a. Keep hands steady and swing opposite legs (both using left or right) across the body—then swing leg out to the side, moving as far across and out to the side as possible.

Breathing. As your leg swings across your body, breathe out, as it swings to the side, breathe in.

Repeats. Repeat the whole movement 10 times, then swing the other leg 10 times.

b. Take a few steps backwards (still firmly holding hands) and lean forwards, bending from your hips. Keeping arms quite straight, twist from the waist aiming towards opposite toes with opposite hands. Then repeat with the other hands and toes.

Breathing. Breathe regularly throughout the exercise.

Repeats. Repeat the whole exercise 10 times.

4a.

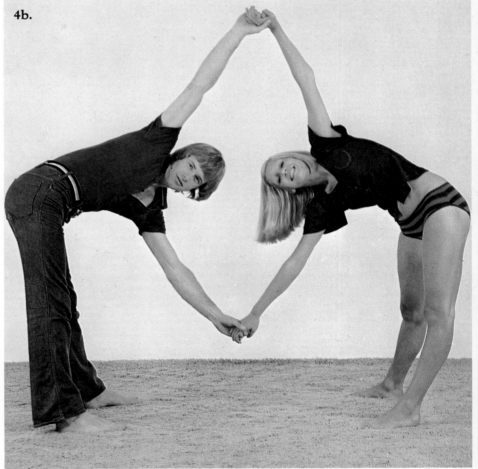

4b.

5. To tone thigh muscles and relieve lower back strain

Lie on the ground, arms by your sides, feet together. Bring your left knee up to your chest and then let your partner press it down as near to your chest as possible—keeping his or her hand firmly on your right knee so that you have to keep your leg on the ground. (Do not force the leg too hard, though.)

Breathing. Breathe regularly throughout the exercise.

Repeats. Repeat 5 times, slowly and smoothly. Now change over and repeat another 5 times with right leg bent.

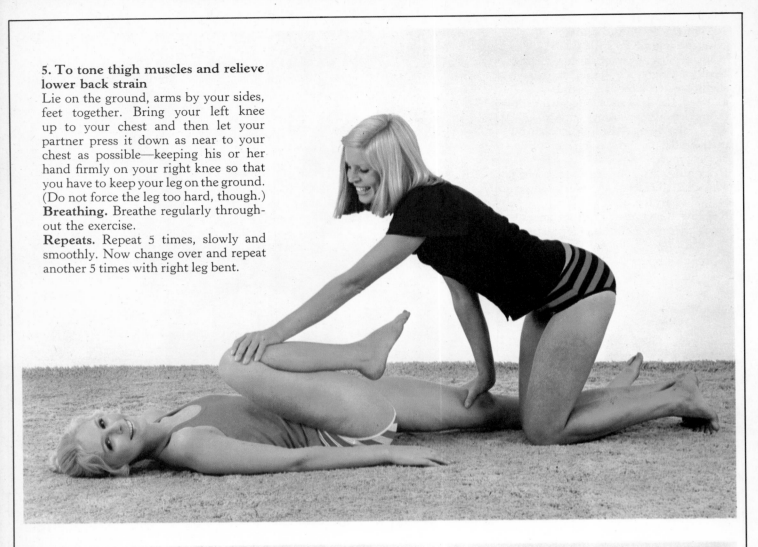

6. To tone thigh muscles and slim hips and waistline

a. Kneel on all fours, head up, palms of your hands flat on the floor. Now straighten your right leg out behind with your toe just touching the floor.

b. Swing your leg (keeping the toe pointed) around to the right side of your body—describing a semi-circle.

c. Then swing it back as far as it will go to the left side.

Breathing. Breathe in as you bring your leg round to the side, out as you swing it back.

Repeats. Repeat the whole movement 5 times, then repeat another 5 times using your left leg.

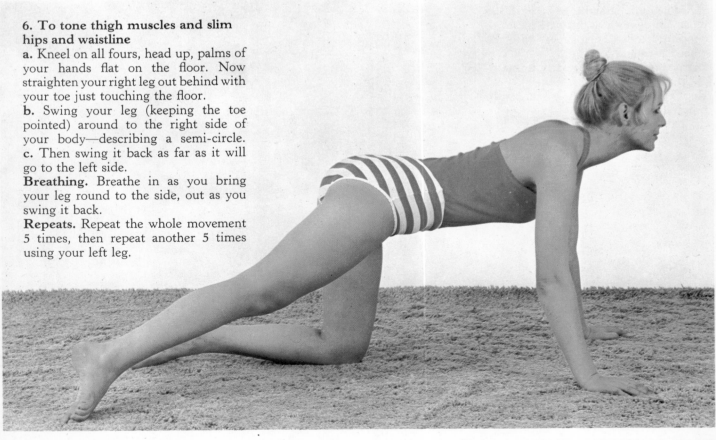

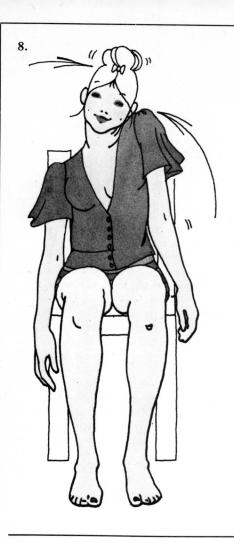

8.

7. To slim thighs

Stand with feet together, arms raised sideways to shoulder level. Now make a small jump with feet together, then kick your right leg up in front of you—keeping the leg and your back straight. Make another small jump with feet together, and then kick your left leg up in front. The completed movement should be rather like very controlled 'chorus girl' kicks—with the legs coming up as high as possible.
Breathing. Breathe regularly throughout the exercise.
Repeats. Repeat 10 times—increasing to 20.

8. To tone shoulder muscles and relieve tension

Stand with your feet slightly apart or sit upright with back straight, on a hard chair. Let your arms hang loosely by your sides. Now raise your right shoulder and try to touch your ear with it. Lower it sharply. Repeat with left shoulder.
Breathing. Breathe in when your shoulder is up, out when it is down.
Repeats. Repeat 10 times, using alternate shoulders. Now raise both shoulders together and repeat 5 times.

9. To pep up stamina and improve general muscle tone

With a partner, stand facing each other and grasp upper arms. Place your feet very slightly apart, with your toes touching your partner's. Now bend your knees to sit on the floor, while your partner is carried forward with the movement. Stand up slowly with the help of your partner. Now your partner should sit while you lean forwards. If possible both of you should keep your heels on the ground throughout the exercise.
Breathing. Breathe in as you sit, breathe out as you lean forwards.
Repeats. Repeat 5 times, increasing to 10 and then 15 times as your stamina improves.

10. To tone stomach muscles, strengthen back and improve posture

Stand with your feet apart, arms straight above your head. Now swing your arms and trunk downwards, trying to get your arms as far as possible behind you through your legs. Now, rapidly bring your body half-way back up and then swing your arms through your legs again. Repeat this movement once more then spring up to starting position again.
Breathing. Breathe in at starting position, out as you 'bounce' through your legs.
Repeats. Repeat whole movement 10 times.

9.

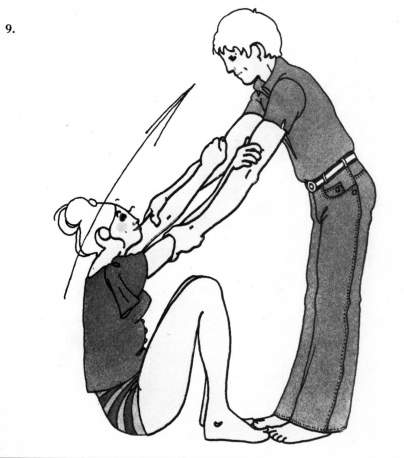

10.

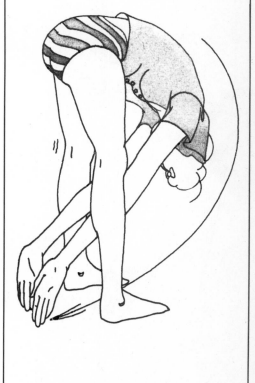

thirty minutes a day work out

This section is intended for those people who have grown used to the idea of regular exercise. The routine is planned to include some fairly tough exercises, so if you still find the Exercises for the fit and lively, pp 104—109, at all difficult do not move on to this set of exercises yet.

Devote just 30 minutes a day to this section, and you will feel fitter than ever before. You do, however, need a certain amount of dedication and concentration. So decide now on the perfect time of day for this half-hour session—and make it a regular part of your routine. First thing in the morning is perfect, but if you cannot steel yourself to get up a little earlier, then set aside half an hour at lunchtime (eat afterwards) or in the evening. Do not be put off by outside distractions—give all your attention to the exercises, and you will reap the rewards of good health, a trim figure and more vitality to bring to leisure activities.

The exercises

Start with breathing, limbering and other exercises as follows:

2 minutes: Stand straight and take deep, regular breaths, filling lungs to capacity and exhaling slowly. Concentrate on good posture (see pp. 72-73) while you are doing it.

8 minutes: Do exercises 1, 3, 4 and 6 from the 'Exercises for limbering up', pages 98-103.

5 minutes: Use this time for exercises 1, 2 and 6 from the 'Exercises for the fit and lively', pages 104-109.

Then progress to the following new exercises:

1. To tone thighs and lower back muscles

Crouch on the ground, feet together, hands resting lightly on the floor. Now spring up, letting your hands swing upwards, and stretching up as far as you can go.

Breathing. Breathe out as you start the exercise, in as you swing upwards.

Repeats. Repeat 5 times.

2. To loosen up your whole body, strengthen back, stomach and thigh muscles

a. Stand straight, feet slightly apart, with elbows bent and hands at chest level, elbows tucked neatly in.

b. Now raise your arms straight above your head.

c. Bend forward and down so that your hands touch the floor, keeping legs and back straight, and 'bounce' hands on the floor three times. Now 'bounce' both hands outside your right ankle three times, and outside left ankle a further three times. Raise your body slowly, bringing your hands back to starting position, then raise your hands slowly above your head. Breathe deeply for a few moments.

Breathing. Breathe in before you start the movement, out as you 'bounce' on the floor and by your ankles.

Repeats. Repeat the whole exercise 5 times.

Included in the first part of the thirty-minute session is (right) Exercises for the fit and lively, 2.

1.

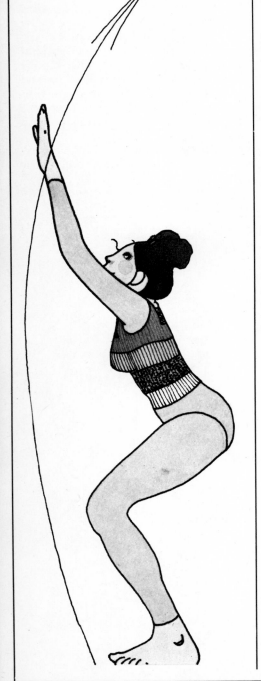

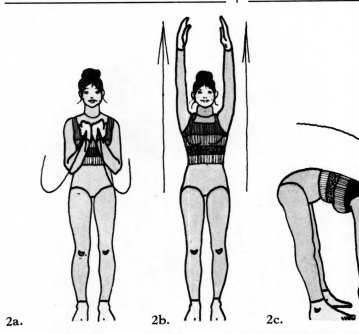

2a. **2b.** **2c.**

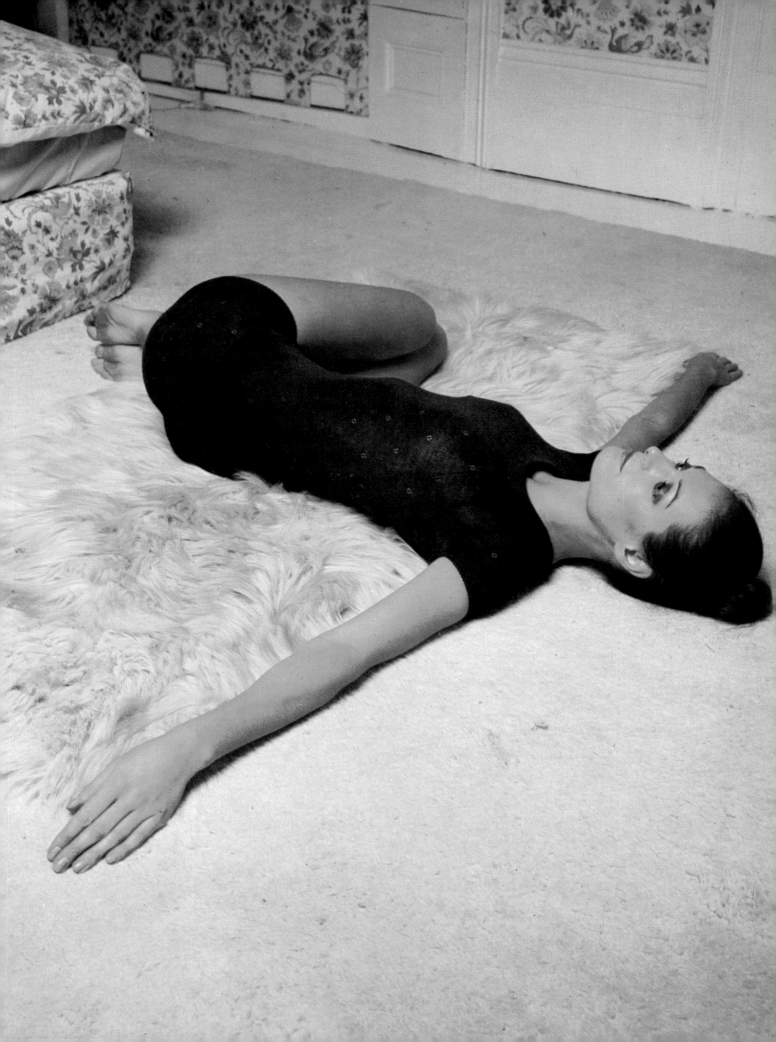

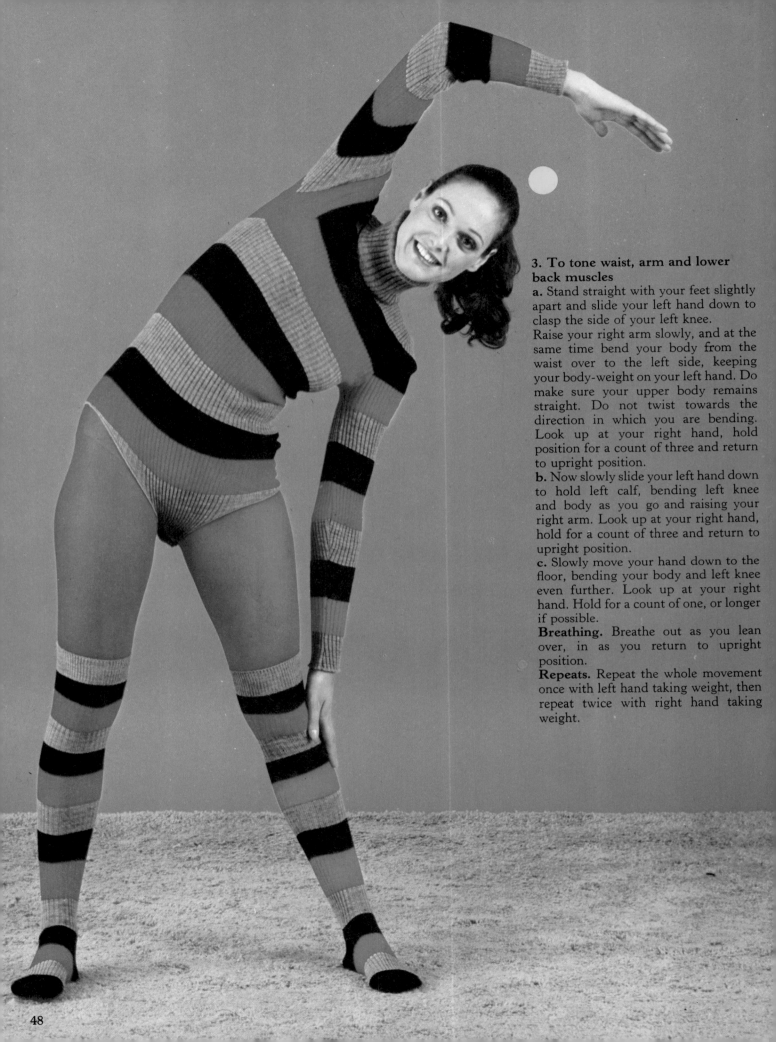

3. To tone waist, arm and lower back muscles

a. Stand straight with your feet slightly apart and slide your left hand down to clasp the side of your left knee.

Raise your right arm slowly, and at the same time bend your body from the waist over to the left side, keeping your body-weight on your left hand. Do make sure your upper body remains straight. Do not twist towards the direction in which you are bending. Look up at your right hand, hold position for a count of three and return to upright position.

b. Now slowly slide your left hand down to hold left calf, bending left knee and body as you go and raising your right arm. Look up at your right hand, hold for a count of three and return to upright position.

c. Slowly move your hand down to the floor, bending your body and left knee even further. Look up at your right hand. Hold for a count of one, or longer if possible.

Breathing. Breathe out as you lean over, in as you return to upright position.

Repeats. Repeat the whole movement once with left hand taking weight, then repeat twice with right hand taking weight.

4.

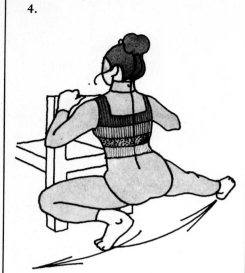

5.

4. To tone calf and thigh muscles
Stand straight, holding on to the back of a chair with both hands, keeping arms straight and feet slightly apart. Now, lunge with your right foot out to your right side, at the same time drop down, bending your left knee out and taking the weight on your left leg. The right leg should be straight and foot pointed. Repeat with the left foot.
Breathing. Breathe regularly throughout the exercise.
Repeats. Repeat 5 times to each side alternately.

5. To firm thighs and stretch back thighs
Sit comfortably on the floor with your back straight. Now bend your right leg in and clasp the instep of your right foot with your right hand, approaching from the inside and bending your knee. Now straighten your leg, raising it slowly toward your right shoulder (still holding your instep). With the leg straight, hold at a fully-extended

position for a count of four, then lower it. If you can only partially straighten and raise your leg just go as far as you can.
Breathing. Breathe regularly throughout the exercise.
Repeats. Repeat 5 times, then 5 times with the left leg. If you find the exercise easy, then repeat a further 5 times raising both legs at once.

6. To straighten lower back, and thigh muscles
a. Stand straight with your feet slightly apart, hands resting on the small of your back.
Now lean backwards, supporting your weight on your hands. Hold for a count of four.
b. Then move your hands slowly down to the backs of your knees, balancing your body carefully. Hold for a count of three.
c. Finally, bending your knees slowly, bend further back and move your hands down to clutch your ankles. Hold this

position for a count of one, or longer if possible.
Breathing. Breathe regularly throughout the exercise.
Repeats. Repeat once only.

7. To strengthen back, stomach and thigh muscles
a. Sit on the floor, back straight and legs together. Now, slowly lean forward to touch your toes keeping your back as straight as possible.
b. Lean back slowly until you are lying on your back then raise your legs slowly —straight and together—and bring them over your head to touch the floor behind you. Hold for a count of two, then lower your legs slowly—still straight—and sit up.
The whole movement should be slow and very controlled.
Breathing. Breathe out as you touch your toes, in as your legs go over your head and regularly until the movement is complete.
Repeat. Repeat 5 times.

6c.

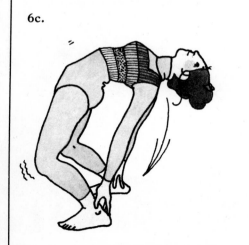

7a.

7b.

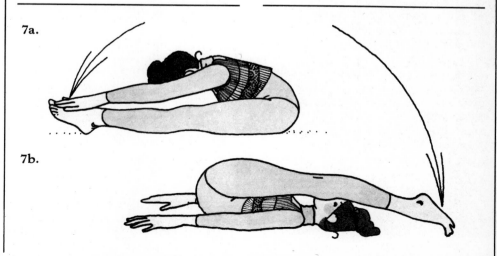

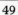

49

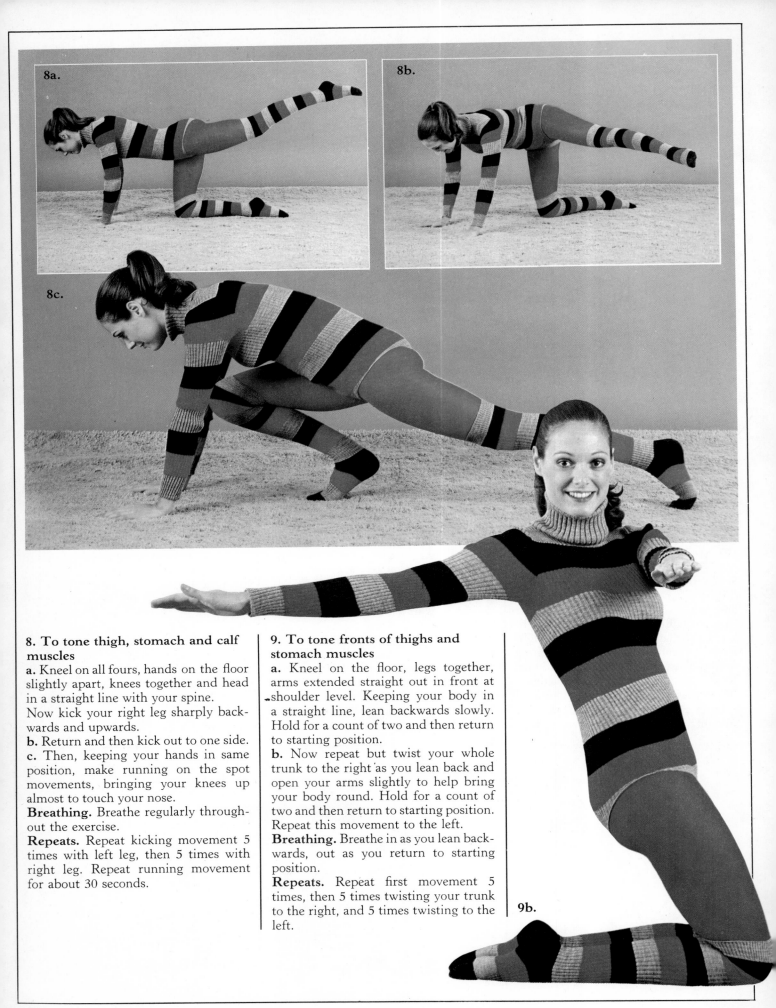

8a.

8b.

8c.

9b.

8. To tone thigh, stomach and calf muscles

a. Kneel on all fours, hands on the floor slightly apart, knees together and head in a straight line with your spine.
Now kick your right leg sharply backwards and upwards.

b. Return and then kick out to one side.

c. Then, keeping your hands in same position, make running on the spot movements, bringing your knees up almost to touch your nose.

Breathing. Breathe regularly throughout the exercise.

Repeats. Repeat kicking movement 5 times with left leg, then 5 times with right leg. Repeat running movement for about 30 seconds.

9. To tone fronts of thighs and stomach muscles

a. Kneel on the floor, legs together, arms extended straight out in front at shoulder level. Keeping your body in a straight line, lean backwards slowly. Hold for a count of two and then return to starting position.

b. Now repeat but twist your whole trunk to the right as you lean back and open your arms slightly to help bring your body round. Hold for a count of two and then return to starting position. Repeat this movement to the left.

Breathing. Breathe in as you lean backwards, out as you return to starting position.

Repeats. Repeat first movement 5 times, then 5 times twisting your trunk to the right, and 5 times twisting to the left.

15. To firm neck and upper arms

Stand straight, feet slightly apart, arms straight out at right angles to your body. Clench your fists tightly and make rapid circular movements backwards with your arms.

For extra effect, hold equal weights in each hand (such as cans of fruit or peas).

Breathing. Breathe regularly throughout the exercise.

Repeats. Repeat circular movement 10 times, increasing to 25.

16. To improve and firm bustline

Lie on the floor on your back with your feet together and hands resting, palms downwards, on the floor by your sides. Now clench your fists and fling hands alternately over your head to touch the floor. Keep up a steady, regular movement.

Breathing. Breathe in as you fling hands over your head, out as you lower them.

Repeats. Repeat 10 times with each hand, increasing to 15.

17. To improve and firm bustline

a. Lie on the floor on your back, feet together. Clench your fists and fling your arms out at right angles to your body.

b. Cross arms alternately over your bust, returning to touch the floor at each side between each 'scissors' movement.

Breathing. Breathe in at the start of each movement, out as you cross your hands over your bust.

Repeats. Repeat 20 times, increasing to 30.

15.

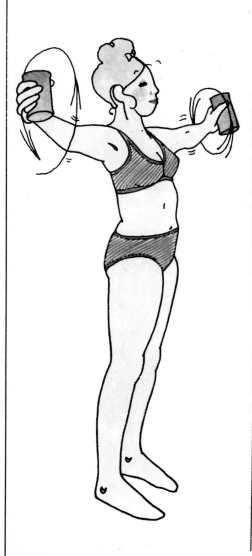

16.

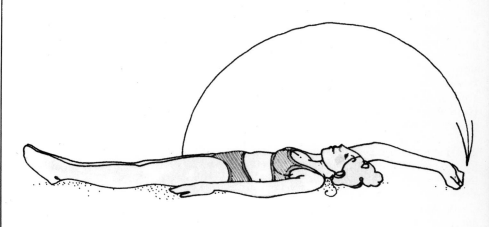

17b.

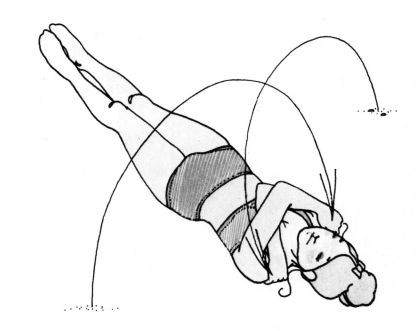

the big build-up

Weight-training is not just a way to build muscle—although it does that very effectively. Using weights forces you to put extra effort into any exercise. And, in the same way that isometric exercises use an immovable object for resistance, the weights provide opposition for the muscles.

A practical weight for women is three pounds in each hand—enough to make the muscles work hard without straining or over-developing them. The recommended weight for men is five pounds in each hand. To build up your muscles and develop a rippling physique gradually increase the weight from five to seven to ten pounds or more when the exercises feel easy. But do not start with heavy weights, you could injure yourself. The weights can be dumb-bells or an equivalent pair of weights which are comfortable to hold. The exercises below are suitable for men or women and we tell you which muscles each exercise will strengthen. Take them easily at first. If you are unused to weights you will probably find that your muscles feel tired after the first session. That means that they are working hard. Remember that it is important to keep a good balance while working with weights, and that all the movements must be performed slowly and deliberately.

The exercises

1. To strengthen shoulders and chest

Sit on the floor with your back straight, legs stretched out in front, arms hanging loosely at your sides with a weight in each hand. With knuckles turned outwards, raise the arms sideways until they are straight overhead. Hold for a count of two and then lower slowly.

Breathing. Breathe in as you raise your arms, out as you lower them.

Repeats. Repeat 5 times, rest and then repeat a further 5 times.

2. To strengthen stomach and thighs

Lie on the floor on your back with feet together and arms by your sides with a weight in each hand. Now sit up slowly, drawing your knees up to your chest at the same time. Hold for a count of two, then lower trunk and knees slowly and relax.

Breathing. Breathe out as you sit up, in as you lower trunk and knees.

Repeats. Repeat 5 times, resting between each.

3. To strengthen hips, back, shoulder and stomach muscles and slim waistline

Stand straight with your feet about three inches apart, holding the weights in each hand by your sides, knuckles facing outwards.

Now swing down to touch your right foot with the weight in your left hand. At the same time the weight in your right hand should swing to the side and upwards. Return to upright position. Now swing down to touch your left foot with your right hand. Do not strain to reach your feet in the first few sessions—you will find that you will be able to do so with practice. And remember to keep your legs straight throughout the exercise.

Breathing. Breathe out as you swing down, in as you return to the upright position.

Repeats. Repeat 5 times each side, rest and then repeat a further 5 times.

1.

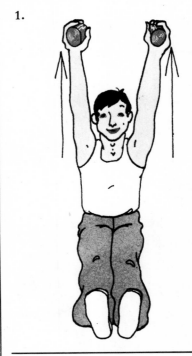

3.

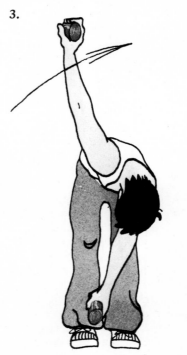

2.

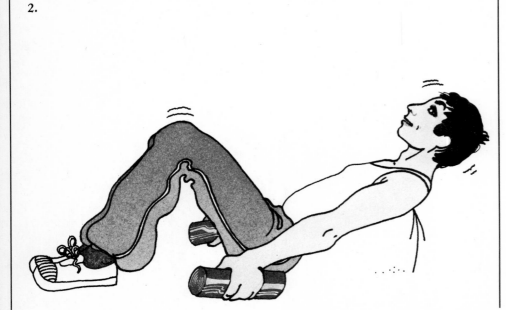

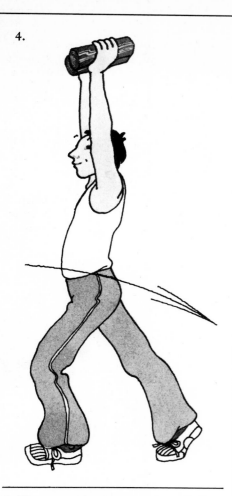

4.

4. To strengthen back, thighs and buttocks

Stand straight with your feet together, arms straight above your head with a weight in each hand. Now bend your left knee and push your right leg straight behind you with the ball of your right foot touching the floor. Now, keeping your arms stretched above your head, change the position of your feet— so that your right knee is bent and your left leg straight out behind you. Stretch your legs as far apart as possible.

Breathing. Breathe regularly throughout the exercise.

Repeats. Repeat 20 times—10 with the left leg forward, 10 with the right leg forward.

5. To strengthen stomach and thigh muscles

Lie on the floor on your back with your feet together, arms by your sides. Hold one weight between your feet. Now raise your legs slowly until they are in a vertical position. Hold for a count of two and lower slowly.

Breathing. Breathe out as you raise your legs, in as you lower them.

Repeats. Repeat slowly 5 times—increasing to a maximum of 10.

5.

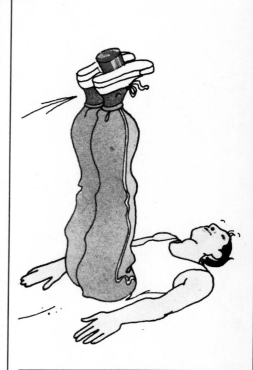

6. To strengthen arm and chest muscles

Sit on the floor with your back straight and legs wide apart and a weight in each hand. Now punch with alternate arms in the direction of your feet, making sure that your arms do not drop below shoulder level. The effort of keeping your arms up despite the downward pull of the weights helps to strengthen the upper arms.

Breathing. Breathe regularly throughout the exercise.

Repeats. Repeat 20 times with each arm, speeding up the rhythm as you go.

7. To strengthen stomach muscles

Lie on your back on the floor with your heels resting on a low chair, legs straight, head and trunk touching the floor. Hold a single weight with both hands.

Now slide the weight smoothly down your thighs to touch your toes, curling your trunk off the floor at the same time, and keeping your arms straight. Return slowly to starting position. (This exercise is difficult, but it is very effective.)

Breathing. Breathe out as you sit up, in as you return to the floor.

Repeats. Repeat twice—increasing to 5 times. Rest for a count of six between each repeat.

7.

6.

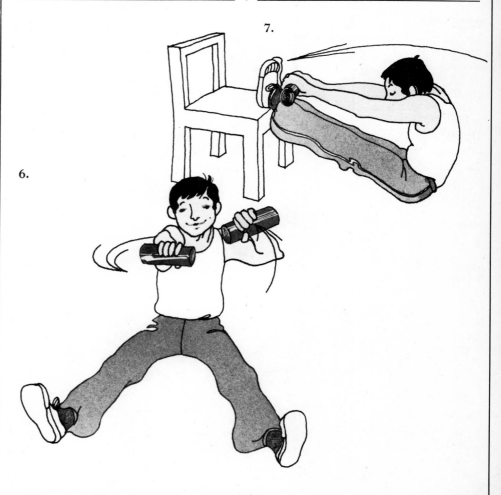

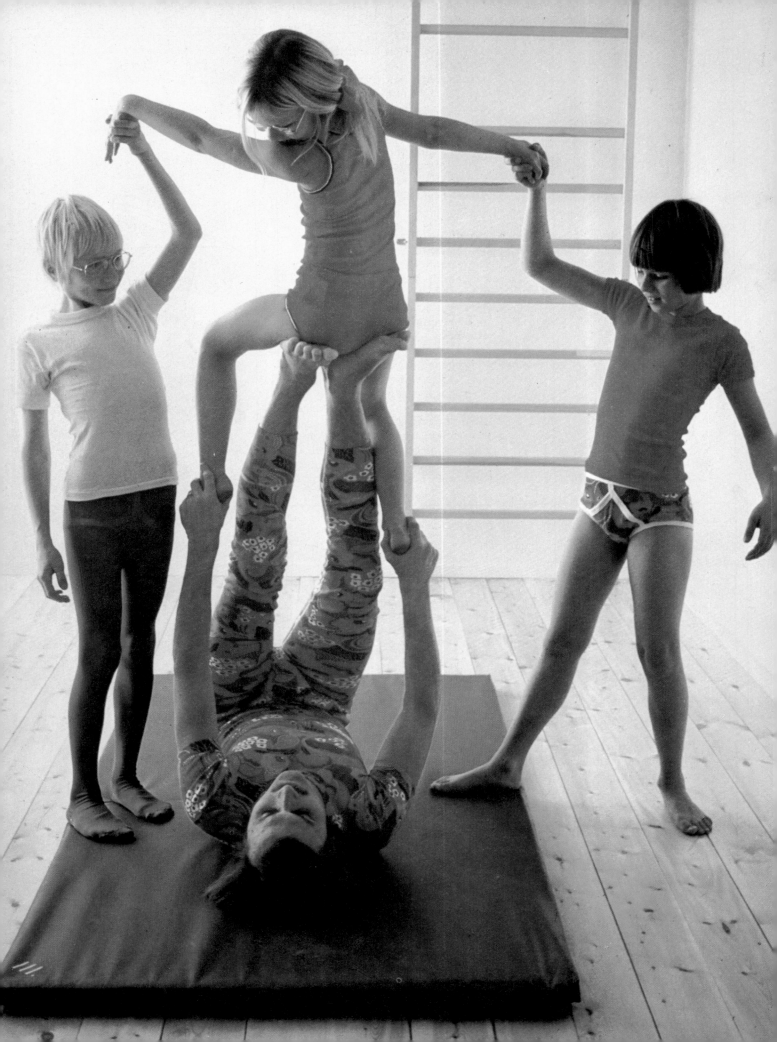

how to stay fit for ever

Keep up some sort of regular exercise programme throughout your life and you will stay fit for as long as you live. The important thing is not to fall by the wayside. However little time you have available, use it to do some well-chosen exercises. Do not let increased domestic or work responsibilities put you off. The more children you have, the more jobs you take on, the more necessary it is for you to be fit enough to cope. Here are some ideas on the kind of exercises to choose for your maintenance programme depending upon how much time you can spare. And remember, when there is really no time to spare, you can keep yourself in trim by practising the isometric exercises—Exercise wherever you go, whatever you do, pages 80-84—or the Exercises in the bath, pages 21-23.

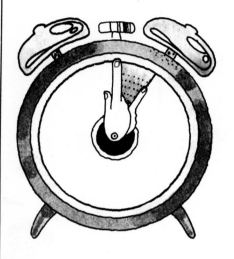

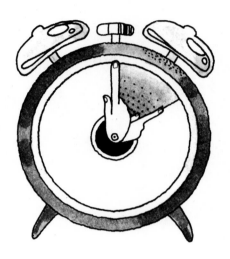

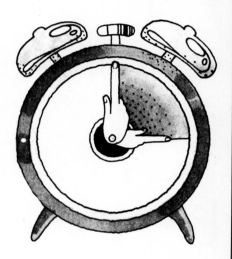

5-minute maintenance programme

1. Start with three uncurling exercises—No. 3 from Exercises for limbering up, page 100—to relieve tension and strengthen arms, back and shoulder muscles.
2. Now whip up circulation with some bicycling exercises—No. 10 from the Thirty minutes a day work out, page 115—which will also strengthen your stomach and back and help to slim hips and thighs.
3. Finally, do exercise No. 1 from the Exercises for relaxation—Yoga, page 90—and rest for a few minutes afterwards if you can.

If you are fit maintain that standard of fitness with exercise and you will find you have more energy to play with, and enjoy being with, your children.

10-minute maintenance programme

1. Start with the tension-relieving uncurling exercise—No. 3 from the Exercises for limbering up, page 100—and repeat the exercise 5 times.
2. Pick one of the following exercises and repeat it 10 times.
For waist and trunk: No. 1 from Exercises for improving problem areas, page 117.
For stomach and thighs: No. 7 from Exercises for improving problem areas, page 119.
For thighs, buttocks and hips: No. 11 from Exercises for improving problem areas, page 121.
For Dowager's Hump: No. 14 from Exercises for improving problem areas, page 122.
For bustline: Nos. 16 and 17 from Exercises for improving problem areas, page 123.
3. Now lie on your back on the floor and repeat exercise No. 6 from Exercises for improving problem areas, page 119, 5 times. This will help to ward off the dreaded middle-age spread.
4. Finally, do a careful, well-executed Yoga pose—No. 1 from Exercises for relaxation—page 90.

15-minute maintenance programme

This is the same as the 10-minute programme above, but you now increase to 10 the number of repeats of your chosen exercise in 2 above.
Then, before doing the final exercise, the Yoga pose, add the following exercises:
Nos. 5 and 6 from Exercises for limbering up, pages 101-102.
Nos. 1 and 4 from Exercises for extremities, pages 95-97.

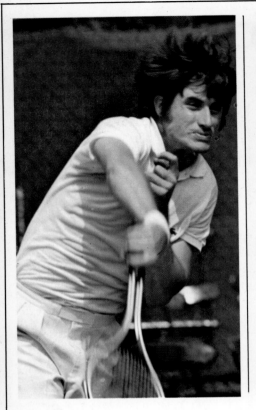
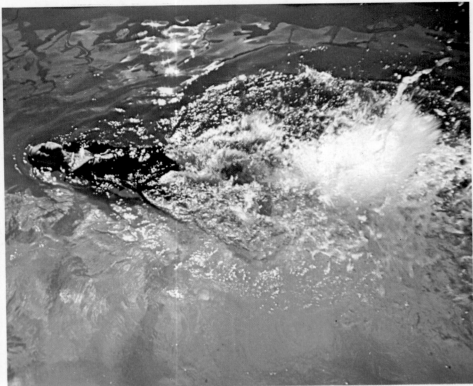

be a sport

Try to back up your keep-fit campaign by exercising regularly in the form of sport. Choose something that you know you will enjoy, and which will do most for your own particular figure problem. (Consult the chart on pages 76-77 to find out which sporting activities can most benefit specific muscles.)

Even summer tennis (however badly you play) and winter squash, played once or twice a week, can help keep you fit and lively. If you do have a weight problem, however, avoid the after-the-game eating and drinking which so often accompany amateur sporting activities. Refresh yourself with water or fresh orange juice—not beer—and avoid those fattening sandwich and cake spreads provided by the club catering volunteers. Below there is a list of sporting ideas to inspire you.

Athletics All branches of athletics are beneficial. You really need to be dedicated to enjoy them, so this is not advisable for anyone who did not enjoy sport previously.

Boxing This is excellent for arms and legs (Deltoids and Calves group) and good for letting off steam. You have to be light on your feet, even if you are a heavyweight, and that may be why

most boxers are also excellent dancers.
Climbing This is good for the single-minded, and exercises arms and legs very well. Psychological make-up is important in climbing—you need to be the calm, resourceful type and have great powers of concentration. Amateurs must not, of course, attempt difficult climbs alone or in bad weather—they can too easily end up stranded.

Cricket or Baseball Standards vary drastically, so pick your club to suit your prowess. It is not a wildly energetic sport unless you are a bowler or pitcher or happen to be in to bat. But it is very relaxing and demands lots of concentration.

Football and Rugby These are both very good for leg muscles and general fitness. The disadvantage is the summer rest between seasons—you must increase general exercise in order to stay fit during the 'off' season. And when you are playing avoid fattening drinks and snacks after the game.

Gymnastics These are marvellous for developing a sense of grace and poise, as well as being good for muscles generally. This is an increasingly popular sport which could be well worth considering seriously if you are fit, agile and have a good sense of balance.

Riding Riding is becoming more and more popular, and it is certainly a good way of getting away from it all. It is excellent for posture and can benefit thigh muscles. The major disadvantage is that it sometimes produces large buttocks.

Skating This is great fun, is good for legs, ankles and general posture and has a definite air of glamour about it, too. It is, however, probably better started young—children do not have so far to fall, and tend to fall less clumsily.

Squash This is good for maximum exercise in minimum time. Forty minutes for a game is usually quite enough. You need to be agile, wiry and have a good eye. Squash is an excellent winter choice as it is played indoors.

Swimming This is another excellent all-year-round sport. Sadly, many adults forget about serious swimming once their school-days are over. But it is a splendid sport to follow with your children, and provides good exercise for most parts of the body—breast stroke, in particular, is excellent for thigh muscles.

Tennis Socially tennis is great fun—but you need to be fairly proficient before joining a club. It provides excellent general exercise, too.